FULL LIFE
FITNESS

A Complete Exercise Program for Mature Adults

Janie Clark, MA

Human Kinetics Publishers

6517327

Library of Congress Cataloging-in-Publication Data

Clark, Janie.
Full life fitness : a complete program of exercise for mature
adults / Janie Clark.
    p.   cm.
Includes bibliographical references and index.
ISBN 0-87322-391-8
1. Exercise for the aged. 2. Physical fitness for the aged.
3. Exercise. 4. Physical fitness.   I. Title.
GV482.6.C58   1992
613.7'0446--dc20   92-2860
                                                                 CIP

ISBN: 0-87322-391-8

Acquisitions Editor: Brian Holding
Developmental Editor: Mary E. Fowler
Assistant Editors: Laura Bofinger,
  Valerie Hall, Julie Swadener
Copyeditor: Wendy Nelson
Proofreaders: Dawn Barker, Laurie McGee
Indexer: Theresa J. Schaefer
Production Director: Ernie Noa

Typesetter: Ruby Zimmerman
Text Design: Keith Blomberg
Text Layout: Denise Peters, Tara Welsch
Cover Design: Jack Davis
Cover Photo: David R. Stoecklein
Illustrations: Kevin Higgs
Printer: United Graphics

Human Kinetics books are available at special discounts for bulk purchase for sales promo-
tions, premiums, fund-raising, or educational use. Special editions or book excerpts can
also be created to specification. For details, contact the Special Sales Manager at Human
Kinetics Publishers.

Printed in the United States of America   10 9 8 7 6 5 4

Human Kinetics
Web site: http://www.humankinetics.com/

United States: Human Kinetics, P.O. Box 5076, Champaign, IL 61825-5076
1-800-747-4457
e-mail: humank@hkusa.com

Canada: Human Kinetics, Box 24040, Windsor, ON N8Y 4Y9
1-800-465-7301 (in Canada only)
e-mail: humank@hkcanada.com

Europe: Human Kinetics, P.O. Box IW14, Leeds LS16 6TR, United Kingdom
(44) 1132 781708
e-mail: humank@hkeurope.com

Australia: Human Kinetics, 57A Price Avenue, Lower Mitcham, South Australia 5062
(088) 277 1555
e-mail: humank@hkaustralia.com

New Zealand: Human Kinetics, P.O. Box 105-231, Auckland 1
(09) 523 3462
e-mail: humank@hknewz.com

To Grant and Bill

Contents

Preface   vii
Acknowledgments   xi

PART I. GETTING STARTED   1

Chapter 1. Getting Fitter Without "Exercise"   3

Chapter 2. Exercise Benefits for the Good Ol' Todays   11

Heart, Lungs, and Blood   11
Muscles, Bones, and Joints   14
Weight Control   15
General Physical Health   16
Mental and Emotional Health   16

Chapter 3. Safety Guidelines for the Older and Wiser   19

Stress Testing   19
Working With Your Doctor   20
Your Exercise Environment   22
General Safety Guidelines   25

PART II. THE WORKOUTS   35

Chapter 4. Aerobics for Keeping Young at Heart   37

You Have Lots of Choices   38
How Hard, How Long, How Often   38
Aerobics for Special Conditions   43
Full Life Low-Impact Aerobic Dance Program   44

Chapter 5.   Muscle Conditioning for Getting Over the Hill (and Over the Next Hill and the Next!)   **57**

Why Work Out Mature Muscles?   57
Types of Muscle Work   58
How Hard, How Long, How Often   59
Muscle Workouts for Special Conditions   61
Full Life Low-Resistance Calisthenics Program   64

Chapter 6.   Stretch Exercise So Joints Don't Get Set in Their Ways   **91**

Types of Stretch Exercises   91
How Hard, How Long, How Often   92
Stretching for Special Conditions   92
Full Life Stretch Exercise Program   94

Chapter 7.   Water Workouts for Staying in the Swim   **111**

How Hard, How Long, How Often   111
Pool Work for Special Conditions   113
Warming Up and Cooling Down   114
Full Life Water Workout Program   115

PART III.   PUTTING IT ALL TOGETHER   **145**

Chapter 8.   Plans and Options   **147**

Chapter 9.   Sticking With It for the Best of Your Life   **159**

Using Self-Psychology   161
Looking at Your Overall Lifestyle   163

Bibliography   165
Index   173
About the Author   179

Preface

Welcome to the Full Life! You are entering an enlightened realm in which mature adults enjoy the benefits of physical exercise while avoiding the fatigue and overexertion associated with many exercise plans.

The secret of the Full Life plan's success lies in putting to use all of the knowledge science has gained from the latest physical fitness research. The result is a program of easy-does-it exercise especially designed not to overtax or discourage you while providing the rewards you deserve.

And those rewards are many! You can improve the health of your heart and discover bottomless stores of energy you didn't know you possessed. If you need to lose weight, you can. And if you need to tone up, you can do that, too. With *Full Life Fitness* you can help protect yourself from the bone disease osteoporosis and from other health problems that threaten our mature years.

In short order, you can expect to start feeling livelier all day through. Before long, family and friends will begin to remark that you're looking terrific. These happy side effects will multiply as you continue to follow the Full Life program. And you can have it all without working too hard or too long.

We know from experience what overdoing it accomplishes. Have you ever known someone who attended an exercise class only to wind up limping around the next day feeling worse than ever? Perhaps the class was simply too exhausting. Or perhaps the workout injured your friend's back, hips, or knees. *Full Life Fitness* drastically reduces the risk of exercise injury, because the Full Life plan has been developed to give you an effective workout without overstressing your joints, muscles, tendons, or ligaments. Where did the notion come from, anyway, that exercise has to "kill" you to do your body any good? It doesn't. And with the help of modern research, this plan has been designed so that you can enjoy all the benefits of exercise while avoiding unnecessary aches and pains.

In fact, if you already suffer from physical problems such as arthritis or back pain, this science-based program can help to relieve those conditions.

Still, science per se can get mighty dry. So the Full Life plan also includes a distinctly human component. Haven't we all embarked on an exercise regimen only to abandon it a short while later? No exercise physiologist worth his or her salt claims that regular physical exercise is such a fascinating endeavor that people should be expected to stick with it effortlessly.

But you can succeed with *Full Life Fitness*, because this program recognizes those special parts of your personality that make you uniquely *you*. The Full Life plan is specifically tailored to satisfy your personal likes and dislikes while meeting your particular physical needs. In this way, it keeps your exercise routine fresh, stimulating, and enjoyable for a lifetime. In fact, by applying the "personal touch" fitness principles that you are about to learn in this book, you should soon come to view exercise as such a pleasant, worthwhile part of your lifestyle that no one ever will be able to talk you out of it!

You probably have noticed that *Full Life Fitness* is not presented as an exercise plan geared only to persons over age 50—or over 65 (or 71½!). That would be absurd. Instead, *Full Life Fitness* recognizes that each person is a little different from the next. Mature adults vary widely in individual matters such as personal fitness level, previous exercise habits, medical history, and state of health.

For example, a clinically obese 45-year-old who has been sedentary for the past 20 years cannot be expected to outdo a healthy 80-year-old who has taken care to remain physically fit and active. In other words, when it comes to aging, we can forget about the numbers! We will achieve a lot more by thinking in terms of physical health, active vitality, and personal enthusiasm for living.

And those are the keys to the Full Life. The Full Life plan provides a flexible routine of gentle conditioning that adapts itself to the needs of mature individuals. So if your circumstances compare with our 40-something-and-inactive example, *Full Life Fitness* can get you back into shape. This is true even if you are already experiencing the medical complications that often go hand in hand with a sedentary lifestyle at any age. If you are in fine fettle, the Full Life plan can help you stay that way. With ease, you can actually increase your fitness level as well as your zest for life!

But what if you fall somewhere between extremes? Let's say that you are in reasonably good health, but you're surely no youngster anymore, and the years seem to have taken their toll on both your figure and your stamina. As a mature adult of *whatever* age or fitness level, you can look to the Full Life program for the answers to your physical exercise needs.

For example, are you looking for extra energy? Would you like to lose weight? Or flatten your abdomen? Perhaps you are interested in stress control. Is it greater flexibility you are after? Or maybe all of the above!

The following pages will teach you how to get exactly what you want from your physical activity program. The Full Life exercise selections have been carefully chosen to present only genuinely *effective* exercises. These exercises have been especially adapted so that you can avoid undue stress and impact when performing them. They are accompanied by precise safety tips and useful advice for maintaining protective body alignment during exercise.

Specific chapters examine specific forms of exercise. This way you will acquire a clear understanding of what is to be gained from each particular method. Aerobic exercise is quite different from stretch, and they both differ from calisthenics. One type of exercise will be best for achieving a given goal, and another type might be better for accomplishing a second goal. You soon will be able to match the items on your physical "wish list" with the correct exercises for attaining them.

With this information—along with your singular knowledge of yourself—you will be able to design your own unique Full Life. But don't worry. You are not going to be left on your own without direction! Each chapter gives specific recommendations. For example, certain exercises are suggested as priorities because they offer more major health benefits than others. And chapter 8 presents several Full Life plans from which to choose. There are 3-day, 4-day, and 5-day plans along with a whole month's worth of suggested workouts and fitness activities.

You can follow one of the Full Life plans provided or use them as samples to help devise a Full Life plan of your own. You should feel free to develop a personal plan, because it is basically a fail-proof task. Remember, *any* activity generally is better than no activity! The only way you could go seriously wrong would be to overdo it. And by following Full Life guidelines closely, you will not tend to overexert yourself.

Guidelines are important in fitness management. But so is another critical element: the *fun factor*. Fun is a vital component of any successful exercise program, and *Full Life Fitness* places special emphasis on experiencing pleasure through movement. Tips for increasing the satisfaction you deserve from your exercise lifestyle are given throughout the text. Tips for *maintaining* interest and motivation are provided in chapter 9.

With *Full Life Fitness*, you can take charge of your personal fitness fate, and you may even gain a whole new lease on living in the process!

Acknowledgments

I want to acknowledge the many researchers, health care workers, and fitness professionals who have contributed to the body of knowledge on which this book is based. Special thanks go to Carole B. Lewis, PT, PhD, for applying her extensive medical training, experience, and knowledge in reviewing the manuscript before publication. Special thanks are also extended to Brian Holding, director of the HK Trade Book Division, and to Mary Fowler, developmental editor, for their invaluable guidance during the project. Appreciation is expressed to Grant Clark for his assistance in recording the manuscript on computer. And warm thanks are offered to all of the mature adults with whom I have had the pleasure to work.

PART I

GETTING STARTED

CHAPTER 1

Getting Fitter Without "Exercise"

Does physical exercise actually reverse the natural aging process? Scientists say no, that would be an overstatement. But the researchers have amassed abundant evidence that exercise aids in weight control, increases strength and endurance, enhances flexibility, and reduces the risk of heart disease and other health disorders. In other words, exercise fights the very things most of us would like to erase about aging: weight gain, loss of stamina, stiffness, and medical problems!

You don't have to be a scientist to see the difference between active and inactive adults. Active people look better, have better health, and enjoy a higher quality of life. Living is just more fun when you're fit. And researchers do agree that being unfit *is* reversible.

So how do we get fitter? Is it necessary to go out and run 9 or 10 miles every other day? No. In fact, that may do more harm than

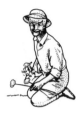

good for many people. Let's take a look at some surprising facts about physical fitness.

First of all, the main problem with today's population is not that we fall short of top-notch fitness but that, as a group, we are almost completely sedentary. A Harris survey of older Americans conducted for the National Council on Aging revealed that 75% of the respondents undertook little, if any, physical exercise. Inactivity, not imperfection, is the enemy.

Slattery and colleagues at the University of Utah medical school recently completed a 20-year study of 3,000 railroad workers. They found that inactive people are at 30% higher risk of coronary artery disease than active persons. And being active doesn't mean that you have to be marathon material. Enjoying light recreational activities such as walking or raking leaves for half an hour a day appears to be sufficient to discourage the onset of coronary artery disease.

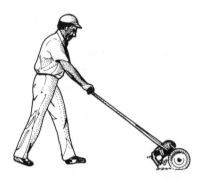

Isn't that fantastic news? For too long, we have been operating under mistaken notions promoted by the "No pain, no gain" school of thought. We were warned that to protect our hearts and extend our lives we must take up long, strenuous exercise regimens, for example high-impact activities like jumping jacks and running. This was presented as an either-or proposition. Either you become an athlete or you die. Most of us were so put off by this intimidating news that we simply turned on the television set and grabbed some potato chips to get our minds off our impending doom!

And there we sit, a society of "couch potatoes." We *are* shortening our lives. Not because we refuse to train for bicycle races and triathlons, but because we aren't moving at all.

Granted, the higher fitness levels achieved through intensive exercise training do produce measurable health benefits. But just for a moment let's think in narrower terms about simply saving lives. Inactivity is a major risk factor for premature death. Moderate exercise, on the other hand, prolongs life. "Moderate" might be defined as including such pleasurable activities as gardening, square dancing, and walking the dog.

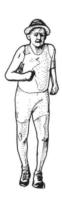

And this isn't guesswork anymore. It has been supported by major research projects lasting many years and studying thousands of subjects. Ekelund and associates' 8-1/2-year study involving 4,276 men found moderate activity to be *substantially* healthier than virtual inactivity. And an investigation by Blair and colleagues at the Institute of Aerobic Research in Dallas concluded that inactive men were 2-1/2 times more likely to die during an 8-year follow-up period than men who were simply moderately active. Prospects for the *very* active subjects of that study were even somewhat better.

But let's worry about becoming moderately active first! That is when the really big health gains show up—when we quit the sedentary lifestyle and take up a moderately active one. This was reconfirmed by a celebrated study led by R.S. Paffenbarger that scrutinized the lifestyles and mortality rates of nearly 17,000 male

Harvard alumni who had entered the school between 1916 and 1950. And similar trends have been found among women.

So let's use this information as a practical part of our Full Life plans. It should suggest that if you are out of shape and maybe less than enthusiastic about starting a structured exercise program, there still is hope for getting back on the road to fitness. Simply bring to mind some reasonably active hobby or pastime you recall enjoying. This could be anything from nature photography to ballroom dance. It might be hunting for shells along the beach or traipsing through sprawling flea markets. How about some sightseeing by bicycle?

Just remember one activity you have had fun at in the past, and *take it up again*. Or participate more regularly. You need not tackle mastering new skills. It is fine to select a familiar activity with which you are already comfortable, something you know you can do successfully. If you prefer, however, you can pursue a new form of recreation that piques your interest. The main thing is to settle on something you'll enjoy.

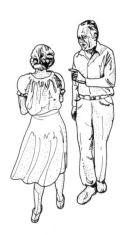

The physical demands of the activity may be quite mild. For instance, one enterprising man named Jack kicked off his Full Life by becoming an accomplished home baker. He resolved to bake a loaf of nutritious, high-fiber bread every day. In this way, Jack improved his diet and increased his physical activity level with all the shopping, carrying, standing, stirring, and kneading involved in his new avocation. Becoming rather an expert at his art, Jack began to get outdoors regularly, searching the countryside on foot for natural ingredients to go in his doughs.

If your lifestyle has been sedentary, give yourself this Full Life gift. Having chosen the gently active enterprise that is right for *you*, devote half an hour a day to it or 1 hour every other day. Stick with it for a month, and then just see if you don't feel keener. At that point, you should undertake a small increase in activity—that is, activity that is equally custom-fitted to you as an individual. The *Full Life Fitness* program will guide you to the forms of movement best for satisfying your personal tastes and goals.

If you feel inspired to increase activity before the first month ends, that is great! But if it takes longer than a month, that is fine, too. Do not take the next step until you feel that you are truly ready. Just continue following your active leisure plan. In due time, you should come to enjoy a new sense of energy. This energy will spark natural enthusiasm for the even greater benefits that can be yours through further movement.

However, if those desirable feelings are slow in coming—or if they never come at all—*do not suspend your active leisure program.* Keep at it! And if you grow weary of one mild activity, then substitute another. Remember, it is the small step you take from being nonactive to becoming moderately active that is likely to make the biggest difference in your overall health and longevity. See Table 1.1 for possible leisure activities.

What if you are sold on the concept of gentle physical recreation, but you are still not sure what type of activity you should try? In

TABLE 1.1

Suggested Leisure Activity Options	
• Walking	• Tennis
• Bicycling	• Badminton
• Sightseeing on foot or bicycle	• Tossing a football or softball
• Window shopping	• Bird watching
• Ballroom dancing	• Berry picking
• Clogging	• Gathering natural supplies (such as shells or leaves) for craft work
• Square dancing	• Photography
• Line dancing	• Collecting (antiques, stamps, or other items that require getting out, walking, and hunting)
• Gardening	
• Raking leaves	• Any active hobby
• Carpentry	
• Golf (walking the course)	

that case, here is a good old standby with which to begin your Full Life. Simply walk a mile every day. If you need to stop and rest sometimes, stop and rest. If you don't make a mile the first day, do your best, and walk a little farther the next. Aim for a total of approximately 9 to 10 miles per week as a reasonable leisure activity goal. When these miles come without effort, you are ready for the next phase.

But the moment you take that very first step, you have already entered the Full Life. It is just that simple. And once you have come that far, you can grow at your own pace and in your own directions.

When you do get ready to expand on your active leisure program—and maybe you are starting out ready—you will have many attractive options. You can add structured aerobic exercise, calisthenics, stretch, pool exercise, or many other leisure activities. Your personal Full Life plan might include some combination of these endeavors. The program you follow depends upon which activities meet your goals while providing the most enjoyment.

When you are living the Full Life, exercise is not some dreary old chore you have to face. In fact, exercise need not be exercise at all! That statement may not seem to make sense at first, but let's just give it a little thought. Jack's bread-baking venture could hardly be described as traditional exercise. Yet he improved his fitness level by adopting that active hobby. By now you may have considered several activities you recall having enjoyed throughout the years. They are all good prospects for your active leisure program. Why did you remember those particular activities fondly? Because they were *exercise*? Unlikely!

Let's take bicycling, for example. When you were a kid, did you hop on your bike thinking, ''Now I am going to elevate my heart rate into the training zone and maintain that intensity level for 20

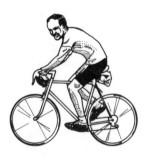

minutes in order to achieve cardiovascular conditioning"? No way! You simply pedaled about shouting hello to your friends, taking in the scenery, and having a good time. You did get your exercise, but the object was to have fun, and you succeeded. Now guess what—it will still be fun!

Put care into choosing an initial leisure activity that will get your Full Life off to a start replete with personal pleasure. Human movement that results in joy leads to additional movement and from there on to greater joys.

With that in mind, you are now ready to further advance your Full Life plan.

CHAPTER 2

Exercise Benefits for the Good Ol' Todays

The upcoming chapters analyze different forms of exercise separately. We will zero in on the specific benefits and how-tos of aerobics, calisthenics, and stretching. But first let's discuss exercise in general. Why bother with it?

HEART, LUNGS, AND BLOOD

You may have heard or read somewhere that a capacity called $\dot{V}O_2max$ (maximum oxygen uptake) decreases as we grow older. This means that our bodies are no longer able to utilize oxygen as effectively during strenuous exercise. Consequently, we may be unable to work as hard or as long as we did during earlier stages of life. This can result from severe respiratory problems, but most of us do not have those. It is more often caused by factors related to the heart. In many people, with age there is also a rise in *systolic blood pressure* (one's blood pressure during the heart's contraction). The good news is that physical exercise can improve the situation significantly.

Exercise increases the size and strength of your heart. In studies of mature adults with high blood pressure, exercise has reduced not only the systolic but also the *diastolic blood pressure* (one's blood pressure when the heart relaxes between contractions). Significantly, exercise also increases blood supply to the heart muscle itself.

With all of that going for it, your heart no longer has to over-exert itself to get its work done. It is able to pump plenty of blood without having to beat so fast anymore. This causes your resting pulse rate to decrease—a good sign that your fitness level is increasing.

Regular exercise reduces your risk of heart disease. That includes stroke, hypertension, atherosclerosis, and heart attack. An active person who does suffer an attack is more likely to survive than an inactive person. The active person will enjoy a quicker recovery, and her or his odds of having a second attack are lower.

And that's not all of the good news. There is some evidence, although inconclusive at this time, that if atherosclerotic fatty deposits have already begun to obstruct your arteries, you can actually *reverse* that with proper health care. A 1977 investigation conducted by Robert Barndt and colleagues found that people who were most successful in controlling their cholesterol and blood pressure levels were likewise more likely to enjoy a regression of atherosclerosis.

But what about that $\dot{V}O_2$max problem? This question has been addressed by a number of research teams, including one led by M.L. Pollock, which reported its findings in the *Journal of the American Geriatrics Society*. Research shows that exercise raises $\dot{V}O_2$max in mature subjects—that is, exercise provides higher energy and more endurance for *you*.

What does exercise do for our lungs? It makes breathing easier and more efficient. With age, there may be a decrease in *vital capacity* (the amount of air you can expel with one forced breath after inhaling deeply). Lungs and connective tissues become less elastic. Respiratory muscles classically weaken and shorten. But these undesirable tendencies respond favorably to physical exercise. Respiration is improved when the muscles involved are

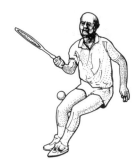

strengthened and stretched. Elasticity is partially restored. And vital capacity increases. Now, that even has a good *sound* to it, doesn't it?

Our circulatory systems benefit dramatically from physical activity. We gain in total blood volume and in red blood cell count. Therefore, more oxygen is delivered to power our cells. Our muscle cells learn how to better extract that oxygen from the blood and how to use it more efficiently for meeting our energy needs.

Exercise decreases the blood's content of cholesterol and triglycerides. With these fatty substances reduced, we are less prone to develop harmful blood clots. The walls of our arteries are less susceptible to that buildup of fatty plaque that can choke off circulation and put us at the head of the line for heart attack or stroke.

But you have probably also learned that there is one special type of cholesterol that seems to protect us from heart disease—*high-density lipoprotein cholesterol*, commonly known as *HDL*. And wouldn't you know it, exercise *increases* HDL.

This was recently confirmed in a study by A.E. Hardman and associates reported in the *British Medical Journal*. Sedentary middle-aged women were placed on a year-long exercise program during which they averaged 155 minutes of brisk walking per week. Although the women made no major dietary changes, their HDL levels rose significantly—so significantly, in fact, that the researchers felt compelled to speculate on what would happen if a large population of women were to establish similar habits. They estimated that the risk of heart disease would have a 54% to 64% decrease over 10 years' time!

Physical activity appears to discourage cardiovascular disease in yet another way. The University of Texas Health Science Center (1990a) reported on an important discovery in men aged 60 to 82: Six months of regular exercise raised the men's levels of *TPA*

(tissue plasminogen activator) by 39%. TPA is involved in the disso-
lution of blood clots. The men's levels of the clot-*forming* substance,
fibrinogen, decreased by 14%.

MUSCLES, BONES, AND JOINTS

We seem to hear a lot about age-related declines in muscular performance. Many researchers have recorded waning levels of muscular strength in older populations. Lean muscle mass has often been
seen to diminish with age. In fact, most of us take it for granted
that our muscles will grow smaller and weaker over the years. But
we are selling ourselves more than a little short with that defeatist
attitude.

Many people become gradually less active as they get older. Their
muscles, suffering from disuse, are subject to *atrophy*. That is, the
tissue shrinks and loses strength. Inactivity almost certainly ac-
counts for more muscular dysfunction than the aging process itself does. And there is an overwhelming body of research showing
that neglected old muscles *can* be revitalized with exercise!

When it comes to the skeletal system, exercise helps to prevent
osteoporosis, the debilitating disease in which bone material thins,
becoming brittle and prone to fracture. Osteoporosis can strike men
but is more prevalent among women. Its painful results may include dowager's hump or dramatic losses of height. And did you
know that one out of every two women over age 75 sustains at
least one fracture associated with osteoporosis?

But here is some remarkable news from the research front: Exercise not only fights the *onset* of osteoporosis, it also helps *rebuild*
tissue that has already begun to grow thin. In a 1981 report, for
example, E.L. Smith and associates described an increase of bone
mineral content in older women given physical activity. Regarding the use of exercise for improving skeletal health, weight-bearing
exercise is effective for enhancing bone mineral content in the spine
and femur, whereas resistance exercise involving the arms and
shoulders affects the upper body.

And exercise doesn't stop at improving bone and muscle tissue.
It also strengthens *tendons* (which attach muscle to bone) and *ligaments* (which connect bone with bone). In this way, exercise stabi-
lizes our joints. That stability promotes unrestricted movement,
and it lowers the risk of accidental injury in everyday life.

Exercise preserves our physical independence and mobility by keeping our joints supple. If you are concerned that it might be too late to regain the ease of movement you once enjoyed, relax! There is plenty of evidence that flexibility can be improved at any age.

And finally, physical exercise can be an invaluable tool in coping with lower back pain, arthritis, and other musculoskeletal complaints. One of the many ways exercise accomplishes this is by improving posture, which can actually ease pain.

WEIGHT CONTROL

The big news in the weight control department is that we can throw out all those miserable starvation diets that seem to remain popular despite mounting scientific evidence that they shouldn't. Far too much emphasis has been placed on diet alone as a means of weight control, and far too little attention has been paid to physical activity. Research shows that regular exercise is essential for making any diet successful in the long run.

But you don't have to visit a research laboratory to know that! Chances are, you have had an acquaintance who achieved quick, dramatic weight loss on some austere diet plan—*and then* soon put that fat (and then some) right back on. A sensible diet and exercise lifestyle could have resulted in permanent weight loss.

As we grow older, many of us complain that we seem to gain weight more easily even though our eating habits have not changed. And no, we're not imagining things! Caloric needs may indeed decrease by 2% to 10% for each decade beyond the age of 20. But that need not create a serious obstacle to good looks and good health. In the absence of any medical condition requiring a prescribed diet, we need only adopt one that is both balanced and low in fat. Good resources for sound advice in this area include your personal physician, a licensed dietician, and your local American Heart Association office.

Equally important is regular physical exercise. Why? Because exercise raises your *basal metabolic rate*. In the simplest terms, this means that, given exercise, your body begins to burn calories more quickly—even when you are resting! Exercise reduces the amount of fat in your body while increasing the amount of muscle. And muscle tissue uses up calories at a much higher rate than fatty tissue does. Moreover, an adequately muscled body looks better and is subject to fewer health risks than an overfat body.

GENERAL PHYSICAL HEALTH

There is some objective evidence that physical exercise may help to protect us from certain forms of cancer. Data collected by Albanes and colleagues in the National Health and Nutrition Examination Surveys suggest that the risks of developing breast and colorectum cancers may decrease with an active lifestyle.

Exercise can play a major role in the prevention and treatment of adult-onset diabetes. It also improves digestion and acts as a natural laxative to help keep us regular. Furthermore, we know that an exercise lifestyle serves us well if we ever need to undergo surgery—because the fitter we are, the lower our operative risks.

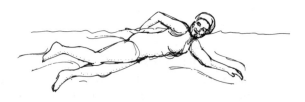

MENTAL AND EMOTIONAL HEALTH

Nothing beats exercise at relaxing the tight muscles that accompany normal, everyday stress. In fact, deVries and Adams's study described in the *American Journal of Physical Medicine* compared the effects of exercise with those of a popular tranquilizer drug. Of the two remedies, exercise provided more relief from the muscular tension suffered by chronically anxious subjects ages 52 to 70.

Material published by Greist and associates in *The Physician and Sportsmedicine* in 1978 supports the theory that physical exercise is useful in fighting depression. Medical guidebooks, such as Gulton's *Don't Give Up on an Aging Patient*, recommend physical activity as a means of alleviating insomnia and irritability. In another text for health care professionals, *Physical Fitness and the Older Person*, Biegel has documented the following benefits of leading an active lifestyle: Increasing physical fitness promotes optimism, improves self-image, and enhances self-confidence. It even appears to sharpen mental ability. Additionally, mature adults who work out exhibit better social adjustment than their sedentary counterparts. In this respect, taking part in group exercise classes can be especially beneficial.

Simply put, exercise helps us to succeed in life and then to fully enjoy our successes. Table 2.1 lists several benefits of exercise.

TABLE 2.1

Exercise Benefits at a Glance

Aerobic exercise is great for
- helping to regulate blood pressure,
- lowering the risk of cardiovascular disease,
- increasing $\dot{V}O_2$max and energy levels,
- reducing total cholesterol and triglycerides,
- increasing HDL (known as "good" cholesterol),
- improving respiration,
- improving the function of the circulatory system,
- controlling body weight and composition,
- strengthening lower body bone and connective tissues,
- possibly offering some protection against certain forms of cancer,
- helping to prevent adult-onset diabetes, and
- combatting mild depression.

Calisthenic exercise is great for
- increasing muscle strength,
- increasing muscle endurance,
- toning and firming muscle tissues, and
- strengthening upper body bone and connective tissues.

Stretch exercise is great for
- improving posture,
- increasing flexibility, and
- achieving relaxation and managing stress.

Note. This chart provides a general overview of major exercise benefits. It is in no way intended to minimize the value of cross-benefits. For example, all three forms of exercise can have positive effects on stress levels and on posture.

CHAPTER 3

Safety Guidelines for the Older and Wiser

Fortunately, statistics suggest that the number of people likely to drop dead as a result of vigorous physical exercise is extremely low. But who wants to be a statistic? Reduce your risk of encountering unexpected health problems by obtaining proper medical clearance before you begin to exercise and by following good-sense safety guidelines in connection with your exercise program.

STRESS TESTING

There has been a good deal of controversy swirling around the use of preexercise stress tests. A typical test involves working out on a stationary bicycle or automated treadmill while a health professional monitors your heart's response to the demands of physical exercise.

Before the test, sensors are placed on your skin to transmit physiological signals to an electrocardiograph machine. The results obtained may then be interpreted, the goal being to determine whether there are any abnormalities in your cardiovascular system. If trouble is identified, further testing can be undertaken to arrive at a firm diagnosis. Ideally, the test should disclose whether (a) you should postpone regular exercise until potential medical problems have been resolved, (b) your exercise plan should be specially adapted to your state of health, or (c) you should go right ahead and enjoy an unrestricted program of sensible exercise.

The problem with stress testing is that the procedure has produced many false results when administered to members of the general population. In other words, a test may indicate the presence of heart disease where none exists, or it may fail to detect disease that is there. For this reason, such testing cannot be practically recommended for just anyone.

However, when the test is given to members of some specific population with a comparatively high rate of heart disease, accuracy increases. Therefore, if you have one or more risk factors for cardiovascular disease, the test can be extremely valuable. You do have a noteworthy risk factor if

- you smoke cigarettes,
- you are 30% or more overweight,
- you have diabetes or high blood pressure,
- someone in your immediate family has developed heart disease or died suddenly for unexplained reasons before age 55, or
- you have a high blood cholesterol level.

Heart disease is relatively common among older populations. For this reason, the preexercise stress test can be a valuable screening tool for anyone age 45 or over, even when risk factors are absent. Whether or not to undergo stress testing should be determined through interaction with your personal physician.

WORKING WITH YOUR DOCTOR

Fortunately, you do not have to complete an independent study of medicine and physiology to make an intelligent decision about stress testing! The best policy is to consult a qualified physician before increasing your physical activity level. He or she will conduct a general physical checkup and then analyze the "big picture" regarding your state of health, your lifestyle habits, and your personal and family history. Your physician is in a position to make an informed recommendation as to whether you should undergo specific testing procedures.

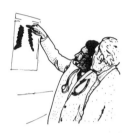

Your doctor can also make useful suggestions about what type of exercise and how much exercise is appropriate to your circumstances. Diabetics as well as persons with asthma, high blood pressure, or other medical disorders are sure to receive special instructions regarding physical exertion. It is imperative that all such medical advice be followed to the letter—and this includes advice pertaining to exercise, diet, medications, other forms of therapy, and, in fact, any matters that may affect one's health.

Ask your doctor to help you set any limitations that should apply to your exercise program based on your individual characteristics. Now is the time—during your preexercise examination—to bring up a chronically sore shoulder, a painful back, that aching knee, or the hip that seems to just give out on you occasionally. Now is the time to discuss what kinds of restrictions an arthritic condition (or varicose veins, obesity, etc.) should place on your activities.

Your doctor can advise you whether to avoid any particular movement that, although fine for other exercisers, may aggravate a preexisting condition in your case. Perhaps performing a limited number of leg lifts will likely benefit an achy joint, whereas too many repetitions might only cause undue wear and tear. Don't be shy! Ask for guidelines and parameters.

For instance, does your musculoskeletal system require the support afforded during a non-weight-bearing activity such as swimming? Or should you work at strengthening your bones with weight-bearing activities like walking or aerobic dance? Is it advisable for you to exercise alone and to take off on long walks by yourself? Or should you work out in a supervised environment? Perhaps a creative alternative would be acceptable. For example, it might be practical to tell your loved ones exactly when and where you will be walking—or to plan a route that calls for circling back at fixed intervals to wave at someone in your household.

In short, *use* your doctor to the fullest advantage. Put to work her or his unique knowledge of your confidential medical history and status. Working closely with your doctor when you plan to increase physical exercise is an important part of the Full Life Fitness program. It helps to *personalize* your workout routine. In this way, you will start out ahead of the game with respect to two vital fitness goals: (a) pursuing the most beneficial forms of exercise, and (b) preventing accidental injuries. Use the Full Life Fitness program as a means of implementing the exercise strategies determined through ongoing cooperation with your doctor.

YOUR EXERCISE ENVIRONMENT

Many elements come into play in achieving a suitable exercise environment. The factors addressed below with regard to choosing a good health club should also be considered when exercising at home.

Floor Surface and Equipment Arrangement

If you are shopping for a health club, look for features that can be particularly valuable to mature exercisers. The floor surface used for group classes should be supportive but "give" a little. A wooden floor with air space underneath is ideal.

Equipment should be positioned to reduce any risk of tripping. When too many exercise machines are crowded together in a small space, the end product can be bumps, bruises, or falls.

Enhancing Sight and Sound

For better visibility during group classes, select an exercise studio that is free of columns and includes a platform for instructors. The room should be well lighted, and glare should not be a factor.

Before you sign up, ask to check the room's acoustics during a regularly scheduled class. If the workout room is an echo chamber, you may have great difficulty hearing exercise instructions. Some clubs offer classes in which only instrumental music is used. It can be much easier to hear directions when your instructor's voice does not have to compete with vocals in the music.

Obtaining Qualified Supervision

Fitness instructors should be certified by a reputable professional agency such as the Aerobics and Fitness Association of America (AFAA), the American Council on Exercise (ACE), or the American College of Sports Medicine (ACSM). *All* legitimate instructors are trained in cardiopulmonary resuscitation (CPR), and the best maintain certification in standard first aid as well. Mature adults should seek out leaders who have also completed relevant specialized study such as AFAA's Senior Fitness training program for instructors.

Setting the Right Temperature

No matter where you work out, temperature is important. The standard recommended range for indoor workouts is 68 to 72 degrees Fahrenheit (although comfort zones may vary somewhat among individuals). Seventy-eight to 84 degrees is a good range for water during swimming pool work.

For outdoor exercise, mild weather is desirable. Research shows that as we get older, our bodies may not release internal heat as readily through perspiration. We may become more susceptible to both hyperthermia and hypothermia. In other words, prolonged exercise in an extreme climate—whether too hot or too cold—is especially inadvisable.

On hot days we should dress in very porous fabrics that allow for the free evaporation of sweat. We should limit our exposure to extreme heat to reduce any risk of dehydration, heat exhaustion, or heat stroke.

As humidity increases, the intensity and duration of exercise must decrease to maintain well-tolerated training levels. This is so because when the air is already saturated with moisture, sweat cannot evaporate as readily into the atmosphere.

Bundle up for cold weather exercise and, again, limit exposure. Cold weather may cause blood vessels to constrict, which, combined with high blood pressure, can strain the cardiovascular system. And keep in mind that extreme cold provides just the right conditions for frostbite. Wearing several layers of lightweight clothing (which can be unzipped and even removed as the body heats up) is usually more desirable than wearing only one or two heavy articles of clothing.

In all types of weather, wear sunscreen to protect your skin.

Proper Clothing

Be sure to choose sturdy, supportive shoes for exercise. The soles should provide plenty of cushion, and the arch supports should be strong.

Do not feel that skimpy leotards or thigh-high gym shorts are required exercise uniforms! Wear the type of clothing you feel most comfortable in. Loose-fitting outfits are best, because clothing should never impede your movement in any way. For some mature exercisers, wearing tights or shorts with snug elastic waistbands can lead to acute discomfort. As already mentioned, exercise wear should in no way hamper the complete evaporation of sweat. Comfortable-fitting sweatbands or absorbent towels can be used to keep perspiration out of your eyes. Both men and women should wear supportive undergarments for exercise.

If urinary accidents are a problem for you during exercise, advise your doctor accordingly. She or he may prescribe medication or suggest specific physical exercises to help increase control. Make an effort to empty your bladder immediately before exercising. Additionally, well-designed absorbent pads (which can be concealed easily under exercise clothing) are available at your local pharmacy.

Water, Water Everywhere

Your workout environment should provide easy access to water. Research suggests that older adults tend to drink inadequate amounts of water in day-to-day life. So remember to enjoy water liberally—including before, during, and after exercise. This is especially important for exercise in hot weather.

Cool water is more quickly absorbed by your system than lukewarm water. Drinking icy water, however, causes cramps in some mature exercisers.

GENERAL SAFETY GUIDELINES

The Full Life Fitness program is all about getting you moving effectively and *keeping* you moving safely. The following rules are important for succeeding on both counts.

Warming Up and Cooling Down

Mature men and women should pay particular attention to the warm-up and cool-down periods included in physical exercise workouts. As we grow older, sudden strenuous exercise can be especially hard on our hearts. Therefore, a healthful warm-up lasting somewhat longer than 10 minutes is in order.

Likewise, abrupt cessation of vigorous work can cause excessive venous pooling in older persons. This means that blood routed to the major muscles of the lower body for exercise energy tends to collect there after the work is done. Having to pump all of that blood back up to the trunk can place unnecessary strain on the heart. But by performing effective cool-down movements lasting somewhat longer than 10 minutes after energetic exercise, we are able to mechanically assist our hearts at this task.

Warm-up Routine.   Instructions for a good basic warm-up routine that should be performed before aerobic, calisthenic, or stretch exercise follow. See Table 3.1 for a sample land warm-up.

For the first 6 or 7 minutes, just walk in place at a very easy pace, allowing your arms to swing gently down by your sides. If you prefer, you can walk about during all or part of this time. For greater variety, include (or substitute) slow pedaling on a stationary bicycle, if one is available. Or dance in a very leisurely, nonstrenuous fashion to the beat of music with a conservative tempo. Simple low-impact dance ideas are given in chapter 4. When used as warm-ups, these movements should be performed slowly and nonvigorously. Later on—during the aerobic portion of your workout—similar movements should be pursued more energetically. That will be the time for higher limb elevations and a brisker pace. But the warm-up is a time for smooth, limbering action. So stick with a very "light" version of all movements.

Continuing your warm-up, spend the next 5 or 6 minutes on rhythmical movements aimed at gently preparing your muscles and joints for greater exertion and furthering the *gradual* increase of

TABLE 3.1

Practical Format for a General Warm-Up on Land

- **Limber up—6 to 7 minutes**
    Good limbering movements include easy-paced walking, slow pedaling on a stationary cycle, and relaxed, nonstrenuous versions of the following movements: the Step-Across (move #6), the Step-Behind (move #7), the Heel-Front (move #8), the Toe-Front (move #9), and the Heel-Out (move #10).

- **Rhythmical exercise—5 to 6 minutes**
    Good rhythmical warm-ups include brief and relaxed, nonstrenuous versions of the following movements: Shoulder Lifts (move #15), Alternate Shoulder Rolls (move #16), Arm Lifts (move #17), Curls (move #22), the Up and Down (move #28), the Standing Cat Curl (move #29), the Shift (move #82), the Quadriceps Firmer (move #110), and the Figure Eight With Foot (move #113). (The Shift [move #82], a water exercise, may be done free-standing on land. The Quadriceps Firmer [move #110] and the Figure Eight With Foot [move #113], also water exercises, may be performed on land by using the wall or the back of a sturdy chair for balance.)

- **Very mild stretching—1 to 2 minutes**
    Good warm-up stretches include very conservative versions of the following movements: the Stretch-Across (move #58), the Upward Reach (move #61), the Chest Stretcher (move #64), the Wall Lower Leg Stretch (move #78), the Good Posture Stretch (move #115), and the Wet Leg-Hug Stretch (move #124). (The Good Posture Stretch [move #115] and the Wet Leg-Hug Stretch [move #124], water exercises, may be done on land by standing with your back to the wall.)

circulation and heart rate. Perform a few repetitions of each movement at a slow to moderate rate of speed. Gently use all of your major joints. The point is to prepare your body so that it will not be surprised later by motions required during your workout. Instructions for standing exercises that safely engage the shoulders, elbows, back, hips, knees, and ankles are given in chapters 5 and

7. These movements are ideal for warming up. During your warm-up, you should perform fewer repetitions and work at a slower speed than you will later during the main body of your workout. Warm up your back with high reaches (move #21) or cat curls (move #29, 31, or 97) before turning or bending your trunk sideways. *Never use weights during your warm-up.* Toward the end of the warm-up, you may include some very mild stretches, but save long, intensive stretches for your cool-down.

Cool-Down Routine. Instructions for a good basic cool-down routine follow. See Table 3.2 for a sample land cool-down.

For the first 5 to 7 minutes after the cessation of aerobic exercise, walk, cycle, or dance very gently as described in your warm-up instructions. Be careful never to drop your head below chest level

TABLE 3.2

Practical Format for a Land-Based Cool-Down After Aerobics
• **Standing cool-down—5 to 7 minutes (longer if needed for heart rate recovery)**   Good standing cool-down activities include easy-paced walking and relaxed, nonstrenuous versions of the following movements: the Step-Across (move #6), the Step-Behind (move #7), the Heel-Front (move #8), the Toe-Front (move #9), and the Heel-Out (move #10). Slow pedaling on a stationary cycle also is appropriate.
• **If you plan to perform muscle-conditioning activities in the same workout, you should take a moment to stretch your calves and hamstrings before proceeding to your calisthenic exercises and then to your final cool-down stretches.**   Use the Wall Lower Leg Stretch (move #78) and the Wet Leg-Hug Stretch (move #124). (The Wet Leg-Hug Stretch, a water exercise, may be done on land by standing with your back to the wall for balance, if needed.)
• **Stretches—5 minutes (or more)**   Perform at least one stretch for each body section listed in the workout instructions of chapter 6.

(that causes some mature exercisers to faint!). Do not discontinue this mild activity until your pulse rate descends to fewer than 100 beats per minute. (We will discuss how to determine pulse rate in chapter 4.) If your pulse rate remains high despite a lengthy period of mildly active cool-down movements, it may be necessary to perform still gentler movements at this time. Such movements would involve conservative standing stretches. In that case, however, the intensity level of the preceding aerobic work may have been too rigorous for you. Next time, devote extra attention to monitoring your body's responses during aerobic exercise. Moderate your aerobic activity, if indicated, to help ensure against overexertion during that phase of your workout.

Continuing your cool-down, spend the next 5 to 7 minutes on sustained, relaxing stretches. Choose at least one activity from each body section listed in the workout instructions of chapter 6. Incorporate relaxing music, if you like. To cool down after a calisthenics-only workout, simply enjoy the stretch routine.

What if you plan to perform both aerobic and calisthenic work during one exercise session? In that case, start by warming up as previously discussed. Complete your aerobic workout. Then perform mildly active, standing cool-down movements for 5 to 7 minutes. Continue this activity until your pulse rate descends to fewer than 100 beats per minute. If it remains above 100 beats per minute, perform the gentler movements as described earlier. Stretch your calves and hamstrings, and then perform your calisthenic routine. End with a stretch routine.

Due to the increased work load associated with supine exercise, some mature exercisers find it less stressful to perform floor work prior to aerobics. People with allergies may prefer to perform floor work before aerobics to avoid breathing any dust that might be kicked up during aerobic work. In these cases, start by warming up. Undertake your calisthenic work followed by a stretch routine. Warm up again, using limbering movements in a standing position for at least 5 to 7 minutes. Complete your aerobic workout, and then perform standing cool-down movements until your pulse rate descends sufficiently. Be sure to stretch your calves and hamstrings at this time.

These warm-up and cool-down instructions are appropriate for both indoor and outdoor workouts. If a stretch-*only* workout is to be undertaken, be sure to precede it with a proper warm-up, as described. Warm-up and cool-down instructions for swimming pool workouts are given in chapter 7. Tables 3.3 through 3.6 provide sample workout formats.

TABLE 3.3

Practical Format for an Aerobic Workout

- General warm-up—10 to 15 minutes
- Aerobic exercise—20 to 30 minutes
- Standing cool-down—at least 5 to 6 minutes (longer if needed for heart rate recovery)
- Stretches—5 minutes or more

TABLE 3.4

Practical Format for a Calisthenic Workout

- General warm-up—10 to 15 minutes
- Calisthenic exercise—30 to 40 minutes
- Stretches—5 minutes or more

TABLE 3.5

Practical Format for a Stretch Workout

- General warm-up—10 to 15 minutes
- Stretches—30 to 40 minutes

TABLE 3.6

Practical Format for a Total-Body Workout

- General warm-up—10 to 15 minutes
- Aerobic exercise—about 20 minutes
- Standing cool-down—at least 5 to 6 minutes (longer if needed for heart rate recovery)
- Stretch calves and hamstrings—1 to 2 minutes
- Calisthenic exercise—about 15 minutes
- Stretches—about 5 minutes

Avoiding Overexertion and Undue Soreness

If you experience any of the following slow-down signs during exercise, severely decrease the intensity level of your workout or simply stop and rest for a while, if necessary:

- Dizziness
- Extreme shortness of breath
- Queasiness or nausea
- Shakiness

If any of these warning signals tends to recur, check with your doctor. And if you ever experience pain or tightness in your throat or chest, stop exercising and consult your doctor immediately. Moreover, see your doctor if you develop any suspicious symptom during or after physical exercise.

Listen to your body during workouts. If you begin to feel exhausted, slow down until you establish a more comfortable pace. Likewise, slow things down if you are unable to carry on a conversation in your normal tone of voice or if your heart rate exceeds recommended levels (as will be outlined in chapter 4).

During calisthenic workouts, you should stop and rest if your muscles begin to burn uncomfortably or if they become so tired that you lose control over the movement of a limb. Remember that muscle tissue will improve if it is worked to the point of feeling fatigued. It is not necessary to work a muscle until it completely gives out on you, and doing so can result in injury. As we get older, it takes longer to recover from tissue injuries, so it is more important than ever to avoid them entirely.

If a certain exercise causes you *pain*, stop exercising and do not perform that exercise again. But remember that there is a big difference between feeling true pain and simply feeling tired. There is also a big difference between real pain and the normal muscular soreness that results from physical exercise. If a movement causes one of your joints to hurt, then omit that movement from future workouts. But if it causes minor discomfort to the musculature *around* a joint, then give yourself a pat on the back. A little muscle soreness is to be expected, and experiencing mild soreness can even be somewhat gratifying!

Often, muscular soreness is more pronounced during the 2 days following a workout than it is immediately after exercise. The best remedy is usually *mild* physical activity. So when you experience normal muscle soreness, take it a little bit easy on yourself during your next scheduled workout, but *do* perform the workout. If soreness occurs on a day for which no structured workout is planned, hasten relief by gently engaging the affected muscles (for example, by walking).

Here are four important Full Life tips for minimizing muscle soreness:

1. Perform a full and complete warm-up.
2. Perform a full and complete cool-down.
3. Work individual muscles only to the point of fatigue, *never* to the point of pain or collapse.
4. Increase your overall activity level only gradually. Adding about 10% more work at any given time is usually enough and is unlikely to cause undue soreness. For instance, if you began your fitness program by walking 10 laps around your apartment complex, increase your activity level by walking 11 laps. Add new work only when your present routine begins to feel easy. If a workout leaves you drained, cut back by 10% and build up again later. Now, you don't have to be a mathematics professor to use this little formula! It is fine to estimate—because, as you can see, we're only talking about making very minor changes as we grow fitter.

When to Skip Working Out

Take a day off from exercise if you have a bad cold or the flu. In fact, take a holiday if you are feeling really run down for any reason. Never exercise when you have a temperature.

Avoid exercise after heavy meals. Waiting for 2 hours is a practical rule of thumb.

It is inadvisable for mature adults to perform vigorous exercise more than 5 days per week or for more than 1 hour at a time. When too much is attempted, desirable training effects do not actually increase by much, but injury rates do.

Taking It Easy on Joint Tissues

Think tall when you work out. Maintaining good posture increases your exercise benefits and can help to prevent unnecessary injuries.

During stand-up work, distribute your weight evenly over both legs. Your feet should be approximately shoulder-width apart (or just slightly farther apart, if that position feels more secure and more comfortable). Your back should be straight, never swayback. Your knees should be relaxed, never locked. You should consciously tighten up your buttocks and your abdominal muscles. You will receive helpful reminders to maintain this posture in the instructions that accompany your Full Life exercise routines.

Paying particular attention to your knees and elbows, protect *all* of your joints, during *any* exercise movement, by resisting the tendency to lock them rigidly. Never hyperextend a joint during any form of exercise. In its simplest terms, *hyperextension* means forcing a joint to overstretch beyond its natural range of motion. *Range of motion* means the mobility or flexibility possessed by a joint.

Do not perform movements at high speed or in an undisciplined manner. Think in terms of *turning* rather than *twisting, extending* rather than *slinging, bending* rather than *jerking*, and *stretching* rather than *bouncing*. Keep your movements deliberate. Work at maintaining a smooth and controlled style of motion.

You will receive many useful reminders regarding safe exercise technique in the instructions that accompany your Full Life exercise routines.

Getting Up and Down During Your Workout

Standing up too quickly after floor work may cause dizziness, which can, in turn, increase the risk of accidental injury. Always take your time in making transitions from the floor to a standing position and vice versa. The same caution applies when moving in or out of a seated position from a chair.

Remember that you can touch a sturdy chair (or other securely stable object) for enhanced balance and support when changing exercise positions.

If one knee or hip is weaker than the other, you can help to protect the affected joint and decrease your risk of falling by using extrinsic support and by favoring the weaker side when lowering or raising your body. For example, to assume a position on the floor, stand facing a stable armchair. Grasp the arms of the chair with both hands. Bend the stronger leg while carefully lowering your body and simultaneously easing the weaker leg onto the floor in a bent-knee position. Still holding the chair, lower the second leg onto the floor and assume a kneeling position. Remove one hand from the chair and place it on the floor, then follow with the second hand. At that point, you will be on your hands and knees. From this supported posture, you should be able to move safely into the desired exercise position. Reverse this process to rise, again favoring the weaker limb and constantly supporting your body with your hands.

At Least Air Is Still Free!

Always breathe naturally and regularly during exercise. You may find it most comfortable to exhale upon exertion and inhale upon release. For example, try exhaling when you lift during a sit-up and inhaling as you lower your body. *Never hold your breath during exercise.* Establish a steady rhythm of respiration in order to furnish your cardiovascular system and muscle cells with the oxygen they need to sustain a beneficial workout level.

PART II

THE WORKOUTS

CHAPTER 4

Aerobics for Keeping Young at Heart

Aerobic exercise is the best form of movement for improving the health of your heart and for controlling (or losing) body weight. In its publication *An Older Person's Guide to Cardiovascular Health* the American Heart Association recommends aerobics as the single most valuable form of exercise for mature adults. This type of exercise conditions bone, muscle, and joint tissue. It is the most efficient form of exercise for improving your serum cholesterol profile, for reducing blood pressure, for increasing $\dot{V}O_2$max, and for raising energy levels.

Aerobic exercise is a *priority* Full Life Fitness activity that you are encouraged to pursue even if you do not perform other forms of exercise.

YOU HAVE LOTS OF CHOICES

You do not have to perform the same type of aerobic work all the time. Good options include brisk walking, low-impact dance, swimming, pool aerobics, cycling, and rowing. All of these activities are reasonably easy on the joints. Stair climbing is another effective option (unless preexisting joint problems increase with climbing). Cross-country skiing is an excellent low-impact aerobic activity. However, due to the potential for twists and falls, it is generally inadvisable to take it up as a novice during advanced years. Exercise machinery that simulates the action of cross-country skiing may provide a safer alternative.

Jogging, running, rope skipping, high-impact dance, and movements such as jumping jacks that require *bouncing* do not spare the joints and may lead to orthopedic injuries in mature adults.

HOW HARD, HOW LONG, HOW OFTEN

Ultimately, your aerobic workout should be intense enough to raise your heart rate into the "training zone." That means you will work sufficiently hard to maintain an elevated pulse rate that ensures major cardiovascular benefits, but you will not raise your pulse rate so high as to endanger your heart by overworking it. The simplest formula for estimating your training zone range is found in Table 4.1.

Subtract your age from the number 220 to find your maximum predicted heart rate for 1 minute. Sixty percent of that figure represents the lower end of your training zone. Seventy percent represents a prudent high-end value for mature adults. Of course, you can obtain more personalized parameters by undergoing an exercise stress test. People taking certain prescribed medications, such as beta blockers, may have lower heart rate values. This formula should be used only with your physician's approval after personal medical factors that might affect heart rate have been considered.

During your aerobic workout, count your heart rate after about 5 minutes of exercise. Do this by feeling for the pulse in your wrist or your throat. Never apply much pressure at your throat, and do not use your thumb when you count. See if you can keep moving

TABLE 4.1

Training Heart Rate Example		
220	160	160
−60 Your age	× .6	× .7
160 Maximum predicted heart rate	96	112
Training zone: 96 to 112 beats per minute Ten-second count: 16 to 18 beats		

at a moderate pace while you check your heart rate. Count for 10 seconds, and then multiply that count by 6. If your product exceeds the upper limit of your training zone, then ease up—you are working too hard. If it falls below your training zone, then try to put more energy into your movements. Check again when you are approximately 10 minutes into your aerobic routine, then readjust your efforts accordingly. With practice, monitoring your heart rate is an easy and effective means of pacing yourself.

But what if you are starting out in decidedly poor shape? Then here is some very good news for you. Recent research indicates that you can improve cardiovascular fitness by working at an intensity level lower than 60% of your maximum heart rate. This is reassuring information. In short, the lower your fitness level is, the less work it takes to improve! As you grow fitter, you can gradually work up to a 60% or 70% intensity level.

Another potential problem is confusion about staying in the training zone. This was best demonstrated by the experience of a woman named Ruth. Ruth told her physician she would like to exercise, but she was then overwhelmed by her physician's instructions. Describing the interview later to a friend, Ruth complained, ''The doctor says I have to subtract this and multiply that, then count this other thing and figure something else! It sounds too complicated.''

With that, Ruth dropped any enterprising notions she had about exercise. What a shame! Of course, heart rate concepts were simple stuff to Ruth's doctor, but they weren't simple to Ruth. And if they seem tedious to you, too, then here is some more good news: *You can go by feel* (see Table 4.2).

Feelings of perceived exertion correlate closely with heart rate values. In other words, if the exercise feels too easy, it probably

TABLE 4.2

Going By Feel
Monitor your perceived exertion level during exercise and avoid the last two stages characterized here, which indicate excessive strain. • "I've just begun, and this is a piece of cake." • "I'm warming up, feeling terrific, and I don't even feel that I am exerting myself." • "I have warmed up, and I feel like I could go on forever." • "Now I can tell that I'm doing some work, but it still feels very easy." • "I'm sweating a little and feeling great." • "I'm sweating more, working harder, and I can tell that I'm getting a real workout. I feel good." • "I'm sweating a lot and working hard. It's difficult, but I can take it." • "This is tough! I'm breathing hard and sweating heavily. I'm not sure how long I can keep this up." • "I am extremely uncomfortable. I'm having trouble breathing naturally and regularly. I cannot carry on a conversation in my normal tone of voice. I feel like I should lighten up." • "I *must* slow down. I never should have worked this hard. Breathing is difficult, speaking impossible. My muscles are aching. I'm exhausting myself, and I feel awful."

is. But if it feels like you're working hard enough to get something out of it, you probably are. If you sense that you're working too hard, that is likely the case.

So if counting pulse rates puts you off, then increase or decrease your exertion level depending on how you feel during your workout. Keep extremely alert for any of the slow-down signals (listed in Table 4.3) discussed in chapter 3. They are strong indicators that you are working too hard.

Generally speaking, aerobic exercise should be performed at least three times a week, spaced out over the course of each week. A beneficial intensity level should be achieved and maintained for approximately 20 to 30 consecutive minutes during each workout. This is an excellent goal to set for oneself. In fact, many highly conditioned mature exercisers enjoy aerobic workouts of greater frequency or longer duration.

TABLE 4.3

Slow-Down Signals
• Dizziness or light-headedness • Extreme shortness of breath • Queasiness or nausea • Shakiness

However, when you are just getting started, it is not necessary to work strenuously for prolonged periods of time to reap physical benefits. You may feel much more comfortable with shorter exercise sessions at first, and that is fine. Just plan an easy schedule and stick with it. You will gradually make gains in endurance. As this occurs, you can lengthen your sessions accordingly. By building up to a 20- or 30-minute aerobic segment in small increments as you grow stronger, you can avoid overexertion, unnecessary injuries, and feelings of discouragement.

You may be shaking your head and thinking, "But everyone knows you have to perform aerobic exercise 3 days per week for 20 to 30 minutes *straight* in order to gain any benefits." Well, that is what we all thought, until recent research findings called these criteria into question. The truth is that aerobic capacity stands to improve with regular 2-days-per-week training periods. However, such training sessions are lengthy, involving the equivalent of covering 3 to 4-1/2 miles in distance per workout. Another drawback with the 2-day training plan is that it does not seem to improve body composition. In other words, the person who completes 4-1/2 miles a workout twice per week is not likely to lose much fat, while the person who completes 3 miles a workout three times per week will grow lean. Both exercisers are doing 9 miles a week, but the more frequent exerciser gets a better return for his or her efforts.

Scientists have documented many cases in which people who trained three times a week for 10 to 12 minutes per workout did, in fact, improve in cardiovascular function. People who hung in there for longer workouts enjoyed greater benefits. But the point is that it is false to say you gain *nothing* from shorter workouts.

For example, a recent study that was well summarized in the *University of Texas Lifetime Health Letter* (1990b) compared two groups of middle-aged men. Both groups performed moderate aerobic exercise 5 days per week. On those days, the men in Group A performed

30-minute workouts, but those in Group B performed three separate 10-minute workouts. At the end of the study, both groups showed significant cardiovascular improvement.

What does all this mean to the mature exerciser? There is much more room for flexibility in exercise programming than was once thought. When it comes to aerobics, you can be *you*. The Full Life Fitness program does recommend that you eventually work up to at least three 20- to 30-minute aerobic sessions per week, if possible. You are also encouraged to shoot for your training zone during those workouts.

However, you should take all of the time you require to reach those goals. Pace yourself below 60% of your maximum heart rate if you need to. Perform short workouts if you cannot tolerate longer ones for physical reasons—or even if you simply don't have the patience for them! If you can't fit a 30-minute session into your day, maybe you can manage three 10-minute sessions. Think in terms of higher frequency if short or easy workouts are necessary. Just do your best. Even if it is unconventional, it will be worth your while.

When the time comes to increase the challenge of your aerobic regimen, the best ways are to work out more often and/or for longer periods of time. Wearing or holding weights during aerobic dance routines is risky for mature exercisers. Increasing speed of movement also is not recommended (except for very minor increases in the briskness of walking, swimming, cycling, or dancing).

Instead, keep your routines challenging by varying your workouts. Add new steps occasionally, and try different combinations of moves. As you become stronger, perform your routines more energetically. Lift your arms and legs higher. Learn to keep moving continuously during each exercise session. Exercise machinery has built-in intensifiers. For example, you can increase the resistance on a stationary bicycle or walk uphill on a treadmill.

And don't forget that you can always *cross*-train, that is, add a totally new form of cardiovascular exercise to your Full Life Fitness aerobic program (or simply substitute a different form for a while). Two useful outcomes of cross-training are that (a) over the long term, it can help you condition additional muscles and muscle fibers; and (b) it can help you stick with your exercise program by preventing the boredom that sometimes accompanies a completely predictable workout schedule. Also, cross-training principles can be applied to forms of exercise other than aerobics. For example, you may vary your active leisure pastimes. Or you might enjoy augmenting your indoor stretch routine by performing swimming pool stretches as well.

AEROBICS FOR SPECIAL CONDITIONS

As previously mentioned, aerobic exercise is the most efficient form of movement for preventing heart disease and for raising energy levels. Instructions on how to best achieve cardiovascular benefits and increase endurance levels have been given.

If your only goal is to lose weight, perform *very* low-level exercise for an hour every day. This means *non-strenuous* activity (40% to 50% of maximum heart rate) that is unlikely to result in excessive fatigue or injury due to overuse. Good examples include casual walking, slow cycling, or relaxed dancing.

Aerobic exercise will be more effective than sit-ups for flattening your abdomen and more effective than leg lifts for slimming down your hips. Calisthenic exercises *are* important for firming and toning flabby muscles, but when the biggest problem is excess fat—and it usually is—high-fat-burning exercises deliver the most dramatic results.

Weight-bearing activity is suggested for the prevention of osteoporosis. Walking or low-impact aerobic dance strengthens the spine, hips, and thigh bones even more than swimming or cycling will. Aerobic dance classes have the added advantage of engaging upper body bone tissue as well.

However, if osteoporosis is already present, weight-bearing activity may be too painful or risky to pursue. In these cases, swimming or cycling (as well as rowing and other seated forms of exercise) may be valuable. Swimming, in particular, promotes ease of movement, decreases the risk of injury from falling, and can condition all four limbs without impact.

Swimming pool aerobic classes offer a viable alternative for many people. One's body does support some weight, but the water's buoyancy gives assistance. Pool workouts also provide a wide variety of movement against water resistance, which is desirable from your skeletal system's point of view.

Aerobic exercise, including dance, can be beneficial to people with arthritis as long as the workouts feature only low-impact movement. Even in swimming pool workouts, the arthritic exerciser should forego higher impact moves. Cycling and other non-weight-bearing activities are enjoyed by many arthritis sufferers, who must exercise special caution to avoid twisting and overstressing joints. A viable way to reduce joint strain is to do frequent workouts of short duration.

Aerobic exercise can be extremely useful in reducing lower back pain. This is because that pain is often secondary to obesity. Excess abdominal fat strains the spine, pulling the lower vertebrae forward and out of proper alignment. Weight loss can restore correct posture and thereby reduce pain immensely.

Aerobic exercise cannot always be recommended for individuals with chronic medical conditions. Regarding asthma, for example, it is well known that aerobic exercise has been observed to spark asthmatic episodes. Therefore, aerobics should be performed only after cautious medical consideration and, in many cases, only under carefully supervised conditions. People with diabetes appear to benefit more from aerobic exercise than from other types of training. The same is true of hypertensives (people with chronic high blood pressure). However, contraindications to exercise and exercise-induced complications are not unknown when these (or other) conditions are present. In *all* cases of medical disorder, it is absolutely essential that an individual work closely with a qualified physician in designing her or his physical exercise program.

Any form of exercise can help to relieve stress and increase mental and emotional well-being. For many Full Life participants, aerobic exercise is the most effective method.

FULL LIFE LOW-IMPACT AEROBIC DANCE PROGRAM

Aerobic dance is growing increasingly popular among mature adults. And with good reason! It meets criteria for safety and effectiveness perhaps better than any other form of aerobic training—not to mention how much fun and social stimulation you can gain through dancing! By sharpening coordination, aerobic dance also offers the adult exerciser an insurance policy against accidental falls and injuries. And it promotes mental clarity by requiring concentration.

The Full Life aerobic dance program has been carefully designed to provide adults with the best features of dance-exercise while eliminating unnecessary hazards. Some older adults perform high-impact training without reported mishaps. However, such workouts never should be undertaken without a prolonged period of gradual and progressive conditioning, and even then they may result in orthopedic injury or contribute to joint damage over the long term. Therefore, in the following plan you will find no instructions for high-impact jumping jacks or high kicks that might harm your hips. There is no hard running or stomping, no twirling around that might cause dizziness. Quick turns likely to damage your knees are absent. And no ankle weights or hand-held weights are used, because they would increase your risk of injury. What you *will* find are simple aerobic steps designed to be both safe and easy to execute to the beat of almost all styles of music.

Much of the choreography in this chapter can be performed while moving forward and backward, to add variety. For example, instead of walking in place all the time, you might take four steps forward, then four steps back. Many of the movements are flexible in this respect. Forward/backward motion can be especially complementary to certain musical selections and thus quite enjoyable to perform.

Be aware, however, that moving backward affects balance in certain mature individuals, increasing the risk of falling. If this caution applies to you, forego backward motion altogether. If you want to "travel," try this simple modification:

Take eight steps forward and then walk in place for eight steps. Turn to face the side, then walk in place there for eight steps. Turn to face the back, walking in place there for eight steps. Then take eight steps back to your starting point. Once there, use the same method to turn any direction you now wish to face.

In this way you will avoid any quick changes that might promote imbalance, and you will always be facing the direction in which you are moving. This technique will go well with almost all musical selections and will safely add variety to your workout routines.

You do not *have* to use music with your exercise routines. However, Full Life Fitness seeks to maximize the fun factor in all physical exercise. One of the best ways to enjoy movement is to perform it in harmony with your favorite kinds of music.

Before introducing tunes, learn and practice your moves without any musical accompaniment. First master the leg movements while keeping your hands on your hips. Then try adding the arm variations provided in your instructions. Finally, select songs of a moderate tempo so that you will never have to work at an unpleasantly fast pace. Your moves should always be accomplished deliberately. The rhythm of your music must allow you to work at a comfortable rate of speed and to maintain complete control over all motions throughout your routine.

Keep things as simple as you like! For example, you might walk in place vigorously throughout your first aerobic musical selection; perform knee lifts during the second; do crossover steps throughout the third; and continue designating just one type of movement per song throughout your entire workout. See Table 4.4.

As you gain confidence and experience, you might experiment with uniting those various movements into simple patterns and

TABLE 4.4

Practical Format for a Simple Aerobic Workout
• **Warm up as described in chapter 3: 10 to 15 minutes**

• **Use 3-minute songs as follows:**
    Song No. 1: Walking in Place (move #1) and Marching in Place (move #2)
    Song No. 2: Low-Impact "Running" in Place (move #3) and Knee Lifts (move #4)
    Song No. 3: Knee Lifts (move #4) and Lift-Kicks (move #5)
    .Song No. 4: the Step-Across (move #6) and the Step-Behind (move #7)
    Song No. 5: the Heel-Front (move #8) and the Heel-Out (move #10)
    Song No. 6: the Toe-Front (move #9) and the Toe-Out (move #11)
    Song No. 7: the Touch-Front (move #12), the Touch-Back (move #13), and Sidestepping (move #14)

• **Cool down as described in chapter 3: more than 10 minutes**

even into combinations of patterns that go with your songs. You can also add other dance movements you know. How about a waltz step, the cha-cha, some clogging, the Charleston, or a gentle version of the twist? See Tables 4.5, 4.6, and 4.7.

TABLE 4.5

Practical Format for a Simple Union of Aerobic Movements During One Song

Instrumental introduction music: Walking in Place (move #1)
Verse No. 1: Knee Lifts (move #4)
Chorus: the Step-Across (move #6)
Verse No. 2: Lift-Kicks (move #5)
Chorus: the Step-Across (move #6)
Instrumental interlude: Walking in Place (move #1)
Verse No. 3: Sidestepping (move #14)
Chorus: the Step-Across (move #6)
Closing Chords: Walking in Place (move #1)

TABLE 4.6

Practical Format for an Aerobic Pattern

4 to 8 counts of Knee Lifts (move #4)
4 to 8 counts of Lift-Kicks (move #5)
4 to 8 counts of the Step-Across (move #6)
4 to 8 counts of the Toe-Out (move #11)

(Repeat for as long as desired.)

TABLE 4.7

Practical Format for an Aerobic Combination

Alternate performing the following pattern with performing the pattern given in Table 4.6.
4 to 8 counts of the Heel-Front (move #8)
4 to 8 counts of the Heel-Out (move #10)
4 to 8 counts of the Touch-Front (move #12)
4 to 8 counts of the Touch-Back (move #13)

(Continue for as long as desired.)

One easy way to increase the challenge of your aerobic workout is to add an extra song for new combinations. Or simply repeat a combination you have developed, using it in two songs of your workout instead of in one song only. Another easy way to increase the challenge is to add an extra song for walking or marching in between songs during which you plan to perform combinations.

Try performing a number of different arm movements during one leg motion. For example, while walking in place, you can reach toward the front or toward the ceiling. Mix and match the arm and leg movements shown in this chapter to discover new matches you feel at ease with. Look through chapter 5 to find additional arm movements (such as biceps curls) that you feel comfortable performing along with the aerobic leg movements given in this chapter.

Try facing different directions while you work in place. You may also enjoy learning to *move* in different directions. We have already discussed stepping forward and backward. Moving on the diagonal is a relatively gentle option. Sidestepping (move #14) involves side-to-side motion, and you will discover that certain other aerobic moves are conducive to lateral motion. Stick with "traveling" that feels 100% secure and natural to you.

Do change music selections occasionally! After a time, you may enjoy going back to repeat "old favorite" dance routines to specific songs.

Begin your aerobic exercise session with a thorough warm-up, and end your session with a thorough cool-down, as described in chapter 3.

In performing your Full Life aerobic movements, be lively! Involve all four limbs. If possible when using your arms, reach for the stars! Remember, however, never to hyperextend (overstretch) *any* joint during *any* form of exercise (as explained in chapter 3). With that caution and all other Full Life safety rules acknowledged, you should feel free to "go for it"!

With the Full Life aerobic plan, you can have fun while promoting good health. If you undertake the program with friends, refrain from feeling competitive. In mature exercisers, feelings of intense rivalry have been known to trigger undesirable autonomic responses—that is, adverse reactions in those physical functions (such as blood pressure) that are not consciously controlled. So, just focus on having a good time! Enjoy any combinations you choose of the following low-impact movements.

Now that we have discussed the theory involved in making the most of the Full Life aerobic exercise program, let's work out!

Low-Impact Aerobic Exercises

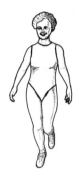

Move #1: Walking in Place
How-To
1. Step briskly, being careful not to walk primarily on your toes. Instead, bring your heel down, also, to touch the floor lightly with each step. This technique provides greater cushioning and shock absorption to help protect your joints during exercise.
2. Try swinging your arms energetically by your sides as you walk.

Safety and Alignment Tips
1. Remember to breathe naturally and regularly throughout this and all of the following aerobic exercises.
2. Remember to stand up tall as you walk.

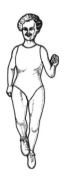

Liverpool
Community
College

Move #2: Marching in Place
How-To
Alternately swing each elbow backward as you march.

Safety and Alignment Tip
Keep your fists loose, never too tight.
Variation
Try marching to the beat of patriotic tunes such as the beloved marches composed by John Philip Sousa.

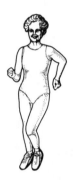

Move #3: Low-Impact "Running" in Place
How-To
1. Instead of lifting your entire foot from the floor as in running, simply lift your heel.
2. Keep your arms active as in running.

Safety and Alignment Tip
Keep your fists loose, never too tight.
Variation
Try this movement in time to merry music with a brisk tempo.

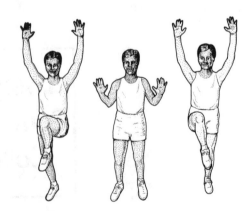

Move #4: Knee Lifts
How-To
Alternate raising one knee and then the other as high as feels natural toward the front.

Variation

If possible, push both arms high with each knee lift. If pain or range-of-motion restrictions prevent high pushes, try pushing arms outward at shoulder level or forward at chest level.

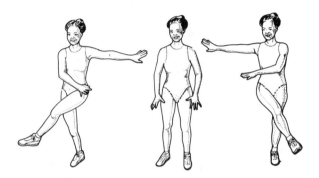

Move #5: Lift-Kicks

How-To

Alternately raise one leg and then the other toward the front. The leg should be partially straight *just short of locking the knee*.

Safety and Alignment Tips

1. No need to bounce or hop!
2. Avoid excessively high lifts.

Variations

1. If this type of lift feels hard on your hips, try sticking with Knee Lifts (move #4).
2. Try swinging your arms back and forth across the front as you perform lift-kicks.

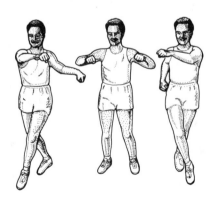

Move #6: The Step-Across

How-To

Alternate feet in touching the toes of one foot in front of the other foot.

Variation

Try adding alternate punches at the front. Punch with the arm op-posite the extended leg. Use a loose fist instead of a very tight one, and be careful not to sling your arms when you punch.

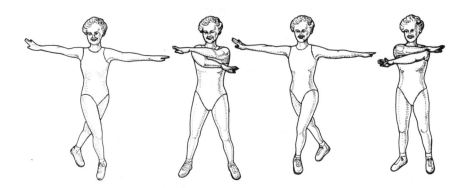

Move #7: The Step-Behind

How-To

Alternate feet in touching the toes of one foot behind the other foot.

Variation

As you perform step-behinds, try adding arm scissors at chest or shoulder level. Alternate arms in scissoring one arm atop the other.

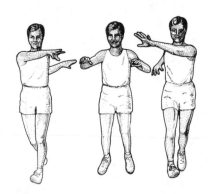

Move #8: The Heel-Front

How-To

Alternate touching one heel and then the other directly to the front.

Variation

Try adding alternate reaches at the front. Reach with the arm op-posite the extended leg.

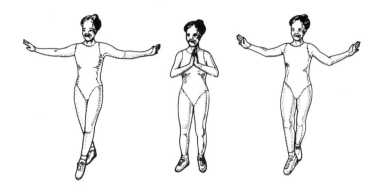

Move #9: The Toe-Front

How-To

Alternate touching one toe and then the other down directly to the front.

Variation

Try adding claps along with this movement.

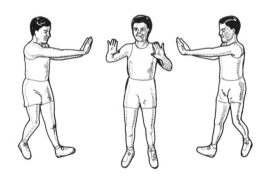

Move #10: The Heel-Out

How-To

Alternate touching one heel and then the other out at the side.

Variation

Try pushing both arms toward the side along with the extended leg. You may turn your trunk gently and look toward the side as you extend your limbs. However, if that type of movement makes you feel uncomfortable or light-headed, substitute pushing both arms toward the front without turning either your trunk or your head as each leg extends toward the side.

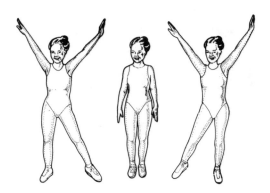

Move #11: The Toe-Out

How-To

Alternate touching one toe and then the other at the side.

Variation

Try adding jumping-jack arm motions. Raise both arms high at your sides as your leg extends. Lower your arms as the leg returns to starting position. If high arm raises are uncomfortable or impossible for you, simply raise your arms as high as feels natural.

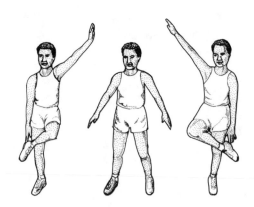

Move #12: The Touch-Front

How-To

Alternate touching one heel and then the other with opposite fingertips.

Variations

1. When touching with one hand, try raising the other hand high overhead. If you have trouble with high arm raises, simply raise your arm as high as feels natural.
2. If you cannot actually *touch* your heel, simply lift it as high as feels comfortable without touching.

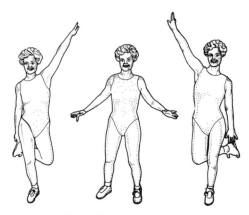

Move #13: The Touch-Back

How-To

Perform this like the Touch-Front (move #12), except touch at the back.

Variations

1. Use the modifications given along with the Touch-Front.
2. Try alternating the Touch-Front and the Touch-Back. First, touch heel #1 at the front and then heel #2. Next, touch heel #1 at the back and then heel #2. Continue alternating in this fashion.

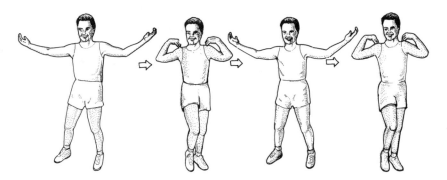

Move #14: Sidestepping

How-To

Take one step to the side with foot #1. Follow with foot #2. Take another step to the same side with foot #1. Follow with foot #2. Now step back to your starting position in the same way but leading with foot #2.

Variation

Try adding shoulder touches along with your side steps.

CHAPTER 5

Muscle Conditioning for Getting Over the Hill (and Over the Next Hill and the Next!)

For the mature adult, muscle conditioning exercises increase both *strength* (the muscle's capacity for maximum voluntary contraction) and *endurance* (the muscle's lasting power).

WHY WORK OUT MATURE MUSCLES?

According to Avers and Wharton's article on age-related changes in posture and musculoskeletal function published in *Topics in Geriatric Rehabilitation*, accidents are the sixth leading cause of death in elderly persons, and falls account for most accidental injuries. This is seldom due to reduction of aerobic fitness but is instead usually the result of musculoskeletal declines. Strengthening exercises help us to preserve the specific muscles and bones necessary for standing and for walking. By developing the conditioning habit *before* old age, we may prevent the falls and loss of independence that have spoiled the aging process for many people in previous generations. Also we may avoid classic inconveniences such as growing unable to get out of cars or up from chairs.

Although weight-bearing activities most effectively fight osteoporosis in the lower body, strengthening exercises involving the arms and shoulders resist development of the disease in the upper body.

Now is the time to begin preventing these predictable potential problems of the future.

TYPES OF MUSCLE WORK

As with aerobic exercise, there are many options for muscle work.

Isometric exercise involves tensing muscular tissue without lengthening the muscle through movement. For example, if you stand in an open doorway and press strenuously against the doorjambs with your palms, this is an isometric exercise. Except for special therapeutic purposes, this form of exercise is not generally recommended for mature adults. It contributes nothing to flexibility, and it can increase blood pressure and intracranial pressure (pressure within the skull).

Workouts with heavy free weights are not recommended for most mature adults because

1. like isometrics, heavy weight work can raise blood pressure significantly;
2. like isometrics, heavy weight work can increase intracranial pressure significantly; and
3. heavy weight work usually causes more injuries than other types of muscular exercise.

An older adult who is *already* conditioned to the use of heavy free weights and who has used them regularly for an extended period of time may well be able to continue safely. However, the heavy-weight lifter should consult a physician to rule out the presence of risk factors (such as hypertension) that would make continuing this practice inadvisable.

For many mature adults, a good alternative is semi-accommodating exercise equipment such as Nautilus machines. This type of equipment usually leads to fewer injuries than do heavy free weights, because it adjusts intensity levels according to the strength of the working muscle. It also permits exercise through a broader range of motion. Still, the mature adult is advised to observe the following safeguards in connection with all strength-training machines:

1. Consult a physician to make certain that personal health characteristics permit safe use of *the particular type of resistance equipment in question.*
2. Work out only under the supervision of a qualified, experienced trainer.
3. Favor a lower level of intensity. Using too much resistance may cause the same questionable outcomes seen with heavy free weight workouts. Fatigue fracture is a particular risk for older exercisers when resistance is excessive. So take a conservative approach to goal setting and to increasing resistance.

The one form of muscle conditioning activity that can practically be suggested for the highest number of mature adults is the *low-weight/high-repetition* calisthenic workout. This type of workout causes few injuries because it is not overly stressful. For the same reason, it is easier to stick with in the long run. It is the most effective method of increasing muscular endurance. And contrary to popular belief, it *can* increase absolute muscular strength in mature adults.

The low-weight/high-repetition workout is unlikely to cause much hypertrophy (muscular enlargement). In fact, as we get older we might reasonably come to expect somewhat less hypertrophy with exercise in general, since neural factors may play an increasingly important role in performance improvements with age. We can, however, confidently expect muscles to tone up, firm up, feel stronger, and serve us more effectively.

HOW HARD, HOW LONG, HOW OFTEN

Once *specific* medical approval has been secured by those wishing to continue or pursue heavy free weight or resistance machine exercise, close supervision regarding intensity, duration, and frequency should be obtained from a competent professional trainer.

For low-weight/high-repetition work, resistance should be such that muscle tissue feels challenged (especially during the final repetitions) but not so great as to make any movement hard to control. It is best to learn exercises without using any weight. As you grow stronger and more familiar with the moves, add weight gradually. You may start out using dumbbells as light as 0.5 or 1 pound per hand. Slowly work up to using heavier weights—from 3.3 to 5 pounds per hand, perhaps more eventually—but never exceed the level at which you can comfortably control all movements during exercise. Reduce the amount of weight you are using if your workout (a) leaves you feeling drained, (b) causes an unpleasant pulling sensation in muscular tissue, or (c) results in sore or achy joints.

Each exercise should be continued until the working muscle feels fatigued. This means that one mature adult may be well served by 5 repetitions, while another may need to perform 25 repetitions or more to get a good workout. You should never work a muscle so long that you experience pain. Instead, persevere only until your muscle feels tired. Then move on to the next exercise in your workout. In some mature exercisers, performing high repetitions may overwork specific muscle groups or joints. In that case, simply limit repetitions to 8 or 16, move on to a different muscle group, and then come back if the first group needs additional work.

Remember, you should never use weight too heavy for the *speed* of your exercise. Excesses in speed or in resistance level lead to flinging, which is traumatic to joints and musculoskeletal tissues.

Use only gentle forms of resistance in high-repetition programs. Hand-held weights are less risky than wrist weights. Hand weights should never be gripped any tighter or harder than is necessary to control them safely. In older age groups, strapping on ankle or leg weights can increase the odds of sustaining an injury. For leg lifts, sit-ups, and push-ups, the weight of your trunk and limbs will supply resistance.

It is not necessary to work muscles in any inflexible order. You may experiment to determine which sequence feels most comfortable to you. Or you may vary the order within your muscle conditioning workouts to prevent monotony. However, proper warm-up and cool-down periods (as described in chapter 3) *are* required before and after every muscle conditioning session.

An optimal training program will include muscle conditioning workouts 3 days per week, spaced out over the course of the week.

Minimal programs include no fewer than two such workouts per week.

Progression for mature adults should be implemented quite gradually. Refer to Table 5.1 for a practical example of how progression might be accomplished gently and safely, and see Table 5.2 for a list of recommended exercises using light weights.

MUSCLE WORKOUTS FOR SPECIAL CONDITIONS

As previously mentioned, resistance exercise decreases the risk of osteoporosis. One ideal strategy for discouraging development of the disease is to perform upper body resistance work in addition to weight-bearing aerobic activity. When weight-bearing exercise cannot be tolerated, skeletal material of the lower body can be engaged by performing activities such as leg lifts, machine exercises, stationary cycling, or swimming.

When osteoporosis is already present to a significant degree, weight bearing is often out of the question due to pain or an increased potential for injury. Likewise, the use of hand weights or other extrinsic forms of resistance during exercise is liable to compromise fragile bone tissue.

One of the best ways to prevent or lessen lower back pain is to use calisthenic exercise to strengthen the muscles that support the spine. For this purpose, pay special attention to

- sit-ups (because your abdominal muscles brace the spine),
- exercises that employ muscles of the shoulder girdle and of the back, and
- exercises that strengthen the buttocks.

The activities included in the Full Life exercise selection are designed to preserve the health of your back. None of the exercises calls for assuming a swayback posture, which can promote injury and pain. Full Life workout instructions also make provision for the proper *support* of your back during physical exercise. Because they oppose each other, equal emphasis is placed on the development of back and abdominal muscles.

People with arthritis can benefit greatly from calisthenic workouts that strengthen the muscles and connective tissues surrounding

TABLE 5.1

A Gentle Progressive Approach
to Resistance Training with Light Weights

First month:
Begin the program by performing 10 (or fewer) repetitions of each exercise while using no extrinsic weight at all. When this routine begins to feel easy, add weights as light as 0.5 to 1 pound per hand.

Second month through 8th month:
Remaining at approximately 10 to 12 repetitions, slowly build up to using 3.3-pound hand weights. Gradually, you may reach or eventually exceed a level of 5 pounds per hand during certain exercises (but *only* the specific movements that you find you can comfortably control using the heavier weights).

Ninth month through 15th month or longer:
Begin increasing the number of repetitions. Do so by small increments of from one to five.

Sixteenth month and beyond:
If you advance to the point at which you are using maximum weight and the addition of more repetitions is not practicable due to time constraints or physical limitations (such as joint overuse or lingering postexercise fatigue), then change your workout. Include new exercises and master variations of old ones. If you like, you can also introduce new forms of gentle resistance: bungee cords for arm and leg work; foam or rubber balls for squeezing activity; dowels and scarves for joint movement. Or you may wish to consider graduating to a workout entailing the use of resistance exercise machines, provided that you obtain appropriate medical clearance and qualified professional supervision.

Note. Some individuals will be able to progress safely at a swifter pace than is outlined in this format, which is mild by design. The challenge should be increased when current activities begin to feel easy.

TABLE 5.2

The Dynamic Dozen
Full Life Fitness exercises with which light weights may be used: Shoulder Lifts (move #15) Alternate Shoulder Rolls (move #16) Arm Lifts (move #17) The Military Press (move #18) The Lateral Raise (move #19) Upright Rowing (move #20) Curls (move #22) The "Muscle Man" Exercise (move #23) Forward Extensions (move #24) Backward Extensions (move #25) Chest Scissors (move #32) The Floor Press (move #35)

affected joints. For example, when arthritis is present in the knee, particular attention should be paid to exercises that engage the front, back, inside, and outside of the thigh. Shin and calf muscles must also be strengthened. The surrounding joints (in this case, the hip and ankle joints) should be conditioned. When arthritis is advanced or painful, no extrinsic resistance should be used during exercise. People with rheumatoid arthritis are likely to perform better during afternoon workouts, when stiffness is less pronounced, whereas people with osteoarthritis may be able to exercise without undue discomfort in the morning. All persons with arthritis should include frequent rest breaks during exercise sessions.

Arthritis sometimes presents us with an exception to the rule that isometric exercise should generally be avoided by older adults. If a joint is inflamed or worn down, calisthenic exercise requiring the limb to bend repeatedly at that joint could worsen the condition. For example, repetitive biceps curls might aggravate an affected elbow joint. Under these conditions, calisthenic work must be restricted to a low number of repetitions. If *no* dynamic movement is well tolerated, an isometric approach may be employed to engage the surrounding muscle while sparing the joint. However, intense versions of isometric activity should still be avoided. An exerciser with an afflicted elbow joint may benefit from pressing the hand *gently* against a wall or tabletop, holding that *mild* press for just a couple of seconds (and taking care to breathe naturally and regularly throughout the activity).

Many people with diabetes can safely and successfully perform calisthenic exercise, but special considerations apply. A person who receives an insulin injection prior to exercise should not work the injection site area. Insulin and/or carbohydrate intake may need to be adjusted to accommodate physical exercise. Readily digestible carbohydrate nourishment should be available during prolonged activity. Any hypoglycemic symptoms arising during physical exertion must be detected immediately. All of these considerations are medical by nature, which emphasizes the necessity of obtaining your physician's assistance in planning and implementing a safe exercise program if you have diabetes.

Balls and bungee cords cannot always be recommended for people with blood pressure problems. If they are used, caution should be exercised to avoid overstraining (which could raise blood pressure excessively). When exercising with hand weights, take care to avoid gripping harder or tighter than is needed to control the weights safely.

As you can see, calisthenics may play a beneficial role in the management of a number of personal health conditions. Muscle conditioning exercise will help an obese person to keep his or her body firm as excess pounds are shed. Also, medically approved calisthenic regimens may be tolerated more easily by some asthmatic individuals than aerobic exercise might be. Finally, the repetition of calisthenic movements can be palliative from a stress-reduction standpoint.

If you have *any* diagnosed medical disorder, you must work closely with your physician to develop and refine a personal calisthenics program.

FULL LIFE LOW-RESISTANCE CALISTHENICS PROGRAM

This program has been especially designed to help mature adults avoid the unnecessary stress, strain, and injury that accompany many other calisthenic exercise programs. All movements known to increase injury risks have been intentionally expunged from our exercise selection.

For example, you will find no deep squats to damage your knee joints; no "hydrants" to compromise your hips; and no straight-legged sit-ups to overtax your lower back. Instead, you will find that only the most natural mechanical angles are employed. Using natural angles makes for a gentler workout—*and* one that is more effective than any workout that permits high-risk positioning.

The Full Life calisthenics program makes safety the top priority. Unlike many other popular plans, the Full Life program helps you to ensure not only that your back is correctly supported during floor exercises, but also that it receives proper support during standing exercise. The Full Life plan promotes the optimal alignment of your spinal vertebrae, including those of your neck.

Another unique feature of the Full Life system is its emphasis on avoiding the stressful *hyperextension* (overstretching) of joint tissues. In performing the calisthenic exercises, remember never to compel any limb to overstretch by forcing it to lengthen unnaturally beyond its limits in range of motion. This precaution applies to *all* exercises. The instructions for the exercises include frequent reminders to avoid hyperextension.

Wherever possible, exercises are depicted in a standing position, because weight-bearing activity advances skeletal strength. Some of the stand-up calisthenic exercises shown may also be undertaken while seated in a chair or on the floor. If you perform seated exercise, take care to sit up tall and straight.

Additionally, the Full Life plan presents exercises that are of special significance to the mature exerciser. For example, there are exercises to condition the forearms and hands (helping to preserve those fine motor skills needed for everyday tasks such as manipulating jewelry clasps, buttoning shirts, and hanging onto drink containers without accidental spills) and leg exercises to strengthen the muscles needed for continued mobility.

Although extra care has been taken in selecting and presenting the exercises, remember that we all differ in personal physical characteristics. If any particular movement feels unnatural, awkward, or painful to you, omit it from your workout schedule.

The use of music during your calisthenic workout is completely optional but is highly recommended for variety and pleasure. Choose tunes with a moderate beat, so that you will never feel obliged to work either too fast or too slowly. Excessive speed leads to flailing, out-of-control movement and ultimately to injuries, and exercise performed too slowly leads to premature fatigue. So select music that sets a comfortable tempo well within these two extremes.

For a balanced workout, warm up as described in chapter 3, and then perform at least one of the exercises given for each body section listed. In time, you may come to successfully perform *all* of these exercises during each of your calisthenic workout sessions, if you desire. Cool down as outlined in chapter 3. Table 5.3 offers a practical format.

TABLE 5.3

Practical Format for a Calisthenic Workout
• General warm-up—10 to 15 minutes • Calisthenic exercise—30 to 40 minutes   Choose one or two exercises for each body region. • Stretches—5 minutes or more

It is important for the adult exerciser to briefly stretch each muscle group after it is worked, before moving on to the next exercise. Doing so helps prevent unnecessary soreness later. This type of stretching is quite different from the flexibility work undertaken during your cool-down period or during a stretch-only workout. At those times, stretches are held for longer periods of time and are performed several times apiece. You will perform such stretches *at the end* of your muscle conditioning workout. But *during* your workout, you need only perform each stretch once and hold it for approximately 10 to 15 seconds before continuing to the next calisthenic exercise. Toward this end, the name and number of an appropriate stretch from chapter 6 has been supplied for each of the following calisthenic exercises. Remember to breathe naturally and regularly during both calisthenic and stretch work.

With that, along with the other safety rules of this chapter and chapter 3, in mind, let's get to work on our muscles!

Low-Resistance Calisthenic Exercises

Shoulder Region

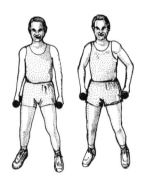

Move #15: Shoulder Lifts

How-To

With or without hand weights, raise and lower both shoulders.

Safety and Alignment Tips

1. Throughout this and *all* hand weight exercises, be careful not to grip your weights tighter or harder than is necessary to control them safely.
2. Remember to maintain the optimal stand-up exercise posture described in chapter 3.

Variation

For variety, this exercise may be performed by alternately lifting one shoulder and then the other.

Stretch

Afterward, perform the Wall Stretch (move #60).

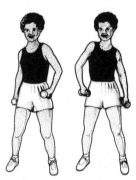

Move #16: Alternate Shoulder Rolls

How-To

With or without hand weights, alternate circling one shoulder and then the other backward.

Safety and Alignment Tip
Remember to maintain the optimal stand-up exercise posture described in chapter 3.

Variation
For variety, this exercise may be performed by circling both shoulders backward (or forward) together.

Stretch
Afterward, perform the Upward Reach (move #61).

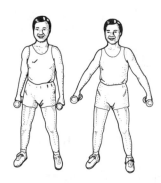

Move #17: Arm Lifts

How-To
With or without hand weights, begin with arms relaxed at your
sides, palms facing inward. Perform small lifts up and down at the
sides.

Safety and Alignment Tips
1. Remember to maintain the optimal stand-up exercise posture
   described in chapter 3.
2. Your arms should be almost straight, but not quite. Do not
   lock them at the elbow joints.

Variations
1. If you have trouble lifting nearly straight arms, lift with your
   arms bent.
2. For variety, this exercise may be performed by executing small
   lifts up and down starting from a low position at the front.
   Also, try alternately lifting one arm and then the other. Or
   try making small circles, rather than lifts, in a low position
   with both arms.

Stretch
Afterward, perform the Big Stretch (move #59).

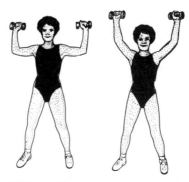

Move #18: The Military Press

How-To

With or without hand weights, begin with arms bent at your sides, palms facing front. Raise your arms straight up, then return to starting position.

Safety and Alignment Tips

1. Mind your posture. Remember to maintain the optimal stand-up exercise stance described in chapter 3. During this exercise, pay particular attention to resisting swayback posture when you raise your arms.

2. When arms are high, take care not to lock your elbows.

Variation

If you have trouble raising your arms high overhead, simply lift as high as feels natural and comfortable.

Stretch

Afterward, perform the Stretch-Across (move #58).

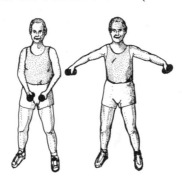

Move #19: The Lateral Raise

How-To

With or without hand weights, begin with your arms relaxed in front of your body, palms facing inward. Lift outward to the sides, then return to starting position.

Safety and Alignment Tips
1. Maintain optimal stand-up posture as described in chapter 3.
2. Throughout this exercise, pay special attention to keeping your elbows slightly bent.

Variation
If you have trouble lifting as high as shoulder level, simply lift as high as feels natural and comfortable.

Stretch
Afterward, perform the Wall Stretch (move #60).

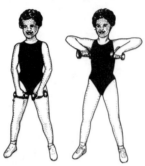

Move #20: Upright Rowing

How-To
With or without hand weights, begin with your arms relaxed in front of your body, palms facing backward. Lift your hands straight upward to chest level, then return to starting position.

Safety and Alignment Tip
Maintain optimal stand-up posture as described in chapter 3.

Stretch
Afterward, perform the Upward Reach (move #61).

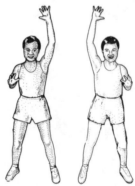

Move #21: Reaching

How-To
1. Without hand weights, alternate stretching one arm and then the other high overhead.

2. Make a point to involve your fingers as you reach.

Safety and Alignment Tip

Maintain optimal stand-up posture as described in chapter 3.

Variations

1. If you have trouble reaching upward (or if you simply desire some variety), reach toward the front at chest level.
2. For further variety, reach both arms upward or toward the front together.

Stretch

Afterward, perform the Wall Stretch (move #60).

Biceps

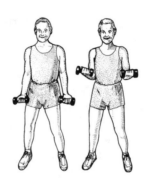

Move #22: Curls

How-To

1. With or without hand weights, begin with your arms relaxed in front of your body, palms facing forward. Bend your elbows to bring your hands upward toward the shoulders, then return to starting position.
2. Concentrate on flexing the muscles of your upper arms as you bend the elbows.

Safety and Alignment Tip

Maintain optimal stand-up posture as described in chapter 3.

Variation

For variety, alternate curling one arm and then the other.

Stretch

Afterward, perform the Upward Reach (move #61).

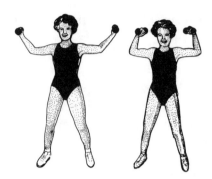

Move #23: The "Muscle Man" Exercise

How-To

With or without hand weights, perform curls (move #22) but higher and at the sides.

Safety and Alignment Tips

1. Maintain optimal stand-up posture as described in chapter 3.
2. Do not overextend your arms at the sides, causing your elbow joints to lock. Instead, relax your arms outward, allowing the elbows to remain slightly bent.
3. Don't be a turtle! That is, don't hunch your shoulders up, burying your neck between them. Instead, keep your shoulders in a low, natural position, and concentrate on holding your back and your neck erect.

Variation

For variety, alternate curling one arm and then the other.

Stretch

Afterward, perform the Wall Stretch (move #60).

Triceps

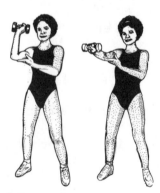

Move #24: Forward Extensions

How-To

With or without a hand weight, hold one upper arm in front of your body with your opposite hand. Begin with your arm bent, palm facing forward. Straightening the arm, press gently toward the front, then raise back to the starting position.

Safety and Alignment Tips

1. Maintain optimal stand-up posture as described in chapter 3.
2. When you press, you may straighten the arm fully—being careful, however, not to hyperextend your elbow joint. During this exercise, remember never to sling the arm or perform the movement too quickly.

Stretch

Afterward, perform the Stretch-Across (move #58).

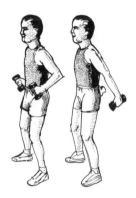

Move #25: Backward Extensions

How-To

With or without hand weights, begin with arms bent at your sides, elbows pointing backward, palms facing inward. Straightening the arms, press gently upward toward the back, then return to starting position.

Safety and Alignment Tips

1. Maintain optimal stand-up posture as described in chapter 3.
2. When you press, you may straighten the arms fully—being careful not to hyperextend your joints.

Stretch

Afterward, perform the Big Stretch (move #59).

Forearms, Wrists, and Fingers

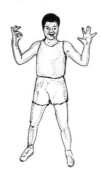

Move #26: Thumb to Fingertips

How-To

Pull your thumb inward to touch the tip of each finger, one at a time, forming a circle.

Variations

1. Although this exercise can certainly be performed in a seated position, perform it while standing, if possible. Doing so helps to strengthen the skeletal system. Maintain optimal stand-up posture as described in chapter 3.
2. For variety, perform with both hands simultaneously.

Stretch

Afterward, perform the Steepling Stretch (move #62).

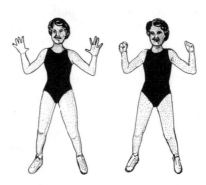

Move #27: Open and Close

How-To

Alternate spreading fingers apart and then making a fist.

Safety and Alignment Tips

1. Follow the posture guidelines given along with the Thumb to Fingertips exercise (move #26).

2. Do not clench fists for more than a second or two at one time before relaxing.
3. Pay particular attention to breathing naturally and regularly throughout this exercise.

Stretch
Afterward, perform the Steepling Stretch (move #62).

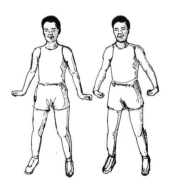

Move #28: Up and Down

How-To
Alternate raising your fist as high as possible and then moving it as low as possible in the opposite direction.

Safety and Alignment Tips
1. Follow the posture guidelines given along with the Thumb to Fingertips exercise (move #26).
2. Use a loose fist, rather than a tight one, during this exercise.
3. Be sure to move only your hand, not your arm.

Variation
For variety, try this exercise with your fingers extended rather than curled into loose fists.

Stretch
Afterward, perform the Turning the Hands Stretch (move #63).

Back

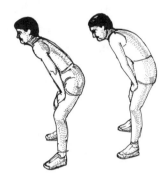

Move #29: The Standing Cat Curl

How-To

Begin by supporting your spine with your hands placed on the front of your thighs. Your knees should be bent, your feet separated for good balance, and your back straight. Round your back upward while contracting your buttocks and abdominal muscles, then return to starting position.

Safety and Alignment Tips

1. When in the starting position, attempt to make your back long and straight rather than swayback.
2. Don't crane your neck. Instead, concentrate on aligning the vertebrae of your neck with those in the rest of your spine.

Stretch

Afterward, perform the Chair Stretch (move #70).

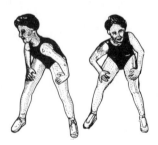

Move #30: Shoulders Forward

How-To

Begin by supporting your spine with hands placed on the front of your thighs. Alternate pressing one shoulder and then the other gently forward.

Safety and Alignment Tip
As with the Standing Cat Curl (move #29), be careful not to crane your neck.

Stretch
Afterward, perform the Chair Stretch (move #70).

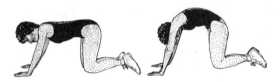

Move #31: The Floor Cat Curl

How-To
Begin with your back straight. Round it upward like a frightened cat, then return to starting position.

Safety and Alignment Tips
1. When in starting position, attempt to make your back long and straight rather than swayback.
2. During this exercise, take care not to lock your elbow joints.
3. As with the Standing Cat Curl (move #29), be careful not to crane your neck. Neither should you twist your neck or hang your head. Instead, maintain a comfortable position confirming the neck as a natural extension of the rest of your spine.

Stretch
Afterward, perform the Leg Hug (move #71).

Chest

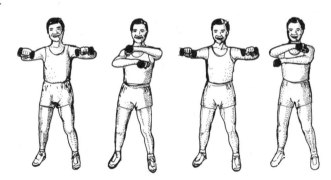

Move #32: Chest Scissors

How-To
With or without hand weights, begin with your elbows bent and pointed toward the back, palms facing downward. Move your arms

forward to cross at the front. Alternate scissoring one arm atop the other.

Safety and Alignment Tips

1. If possible, keep your hands and elbows at shoulder level during this exercise. However, if that position feels too strenuous, simply perform the exercise with elbows lowered. Instead of scissoring, move your arms forward until your hands come near each other without crossing or touching.
2. Maintain good stand-up posture as described in chapter 3.
3. As in the ''Muscle Man'' Exercise (move #23), don't be a turtle!

Stretch

Afterward, perform the Chest Stretcher (move #64).

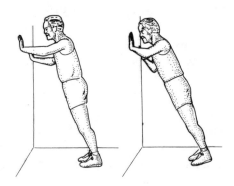

Move #33: Wall Push-Ups

How-To

Stand away from the wall with your arms and legs almost straight but still slightly relaxed at the elbow and knee joints. Bending your elbows, allow your body to lean inward toward the wall, then push against the wall to return to starting position.

Safety and Alignment Tip

Instead of letting your back sag into a swayback position, keep it straight throughout this exercise.

Stretch

Afterward, perform the Chest Stretcher (move #64).

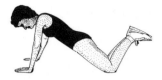

Move #34: The Bent Knee Push-Up

How-To

To reduce stress on the back, perform floor push-ups on bent knees rather than with legs straight.

Safety and Alignment Tips

1. Try to keep your back straight during this exercise. If that feels too strenuous, it is better to raise your hips and round your back slightly upward than to allow it to sag into a swayback position.
2. When you lift the body, do not straighten your arms so much that their elbow joints lock.

Variation

If push-ups strain your wrists, stick with the less stressful chest exercises shown.

Stretch

Afterward, perform the Bent Stretch (move #65).

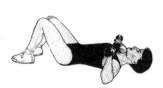 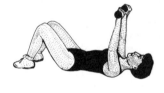

Move #35: The Floor Press

How-To

With or without hand weights, lie on your back with your knees bent, your elbows bent, and your hands at chest level, palms facing forward. Raise your arms straight up, then lower them to starting position.

Safety and Alignment Tips

1. When extending your arms upward, do not lock your elbows.
2. As previously mentioned, you should avoid overgripping when working with weights. At the same time, do make certain that your hold is secure. You certainly would not want to drop a weight on yourself!

Stretch

Afterward, perform the Shoulder-Touch Stretch (move #66).

The Upper and Middle Abdominal Region

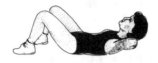

Move #36: The Modified Sit-Up

How-To

With your knees slightly bent, smoothly roll your upper body forward at a moderate rate of speed. Raise just high enough for your shoulder blades to clear the floor, then ease back down.

Safety and Alignment Tips

1. To begin, don't just fall backward onto the floor from a seated position. Instead, use your arms to support your body as you first turn to lie on your side and then gently roll onto your back.

2. During sit-ups, protect your lower back by keeping it pressed securely to the floor.

3. Placing both hands behind your neck provides your head and neck with extra support. To avoid having a sore neck later, be careful not to yank your head up with your arms. Keep both elbows out of sight at your sides instead of pointed upward, and let your abdominal musculature do the work for you. People with dowager's hump syndrome may have a tendency to hunch the shoulders toward the chest during sit-ups performed with hands behind the head. This could contribute to furthering the condition. In that case, swimming pool exercises for the midsection may provide a viable alternative to sit-ups.

4. Many exercisers tend to hold their breath accidentally during sit-ups. You should try to draw the abdomen flat as you work, but don't forget to breathe as you do so! Try exhaling as you lift and inhaling as you ease downward. Breathe with a natural and regular rhythm.

5. Remember not to lift too high and never to perform sit-ups with your legs straight.

Stretch

Afterward, perform the Full Body Stretch (move #68).

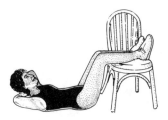

Move #37: The Chair Sit-Up

How-To
For an easier sit-up (or for variety's sake), rest your lower legs on the seat of a chair.

Safety and Alignment Tip
Observe the safety tips recommended along with the Modified Sit-Up (move #36).

Stretch
Afterward, perform the Midsection Stretch (move #67).

Sides of the Abdomen

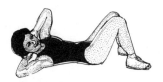

Move #38: The Diagonal Sit-Up

How-To
Bear toward the sides during sit-ups.

Safety and Alignment Tip
Observe the safety tips for the Modified Sit-Up (move #36).

Variation
For an easier sit-up (or for variety's sake), perform diagonal sit-ups with your lower legs on the seat of a chair as pictured in the Chair Sit-Up (move #37).

Stretch
Afterward, perform the One-Side-at-a-Time Stretch (move #69).

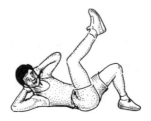

Move #39: The Diagonal Sit-Up with Leg Lifted

How-To

Perform diagonal sit-ups, directing your elbow toward the opposite knee as you hold your leg above the body.

Safety and Alignment Tips

1. It is not necessary to *touch* the elbow to your knee. Lift only as high as feels natural to you.
2. Keep the raised leg relaxed at the knee. Be sure to hold it in *over* your torso.
3. Observe the other safety tips for the Modified Sit-Up (move #36).

Stretch

Afterward, perform the One-Side-at-a-Time Stretch (move #69).

Lower Abdominal Region

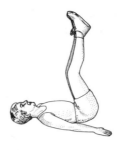

Move #40: Bottoms Up

How-To

Lie on your back with your palms on the floor at your sides and with your legs held above your body. Without swinging or rocking your legs, lift your buttocks straight up off the floor, then return to starting position.

Safety and Alignment Tips

1. Don't try to lift very high. An inch or so is high enough.
2. Remember to keep your knees relaxed.

3. Don't let your feet get away from you. Be sure to keep your legs in *over* the torso.

Stretch
Afterward, perform the Full Body Stretch (move #68).

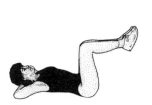 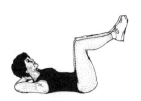 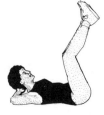

Move #41: The Modified V-Up

How-To
Lie on your back with your hands behind your head and your legs bent at a right angle. Lift your head and shoulders slightly, as in the Modified Sit-Up (move #36). Then lift your feet to straighten your legs just short of locking your knees. Return to starting position by first lowering your head and shoulders, then lowering your feet.

Safety and Alignment Tips
1. As in Bottoms Up (move #40), don't let your feet get away from you.
2. Pay special attention to breathing naturally and regularly during this exercise.
3. Most mature exercisers can safely and successfully perform this gentler, adapted version of the traditional V-up. However, if your back is quite weak or if you experience back strain with this exercise, omit it from your workout schedule.

Stretch
Afterward, perform the Full Body Stretch (move #68).

Hamstrings and Buttocks

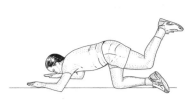 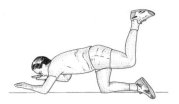

Move #42: The Back-of-Thigh Lift

How-To
Perform leg lifts with the knee bent.

Safety and Alignment Tips

1. Performing lifts with a bent limb reduces stress (as compared to lifting a straightened limb). Do not exaggerate this bend, however, as that might strain your knee. If you feel a pulling sensation in or around your knee during the lifts, you are probably overbending your leg.

2. Placing your elbows on the floor helps prevent undue stress on your back by promoting straight spinal alignment. To maintain an optimal position, avoid excessively high lifts. Keep your neck lined up with the rest of your spine (rather than either craning your neck or hanging your head downward).

3. This is one of those exercises during which some people tend to fling the leg up in a hazardous manner—especially when they grow tired. Remember to execute deliberate, controlled lifts. If you get too tired to perform ''clean'' lifts, take a stretch break.

Stretch

Afterward, perform the Leg Hug (move #71).

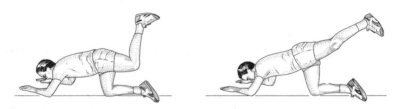

Move #43: Bend and Extend Backward

How-To

Alternate bending and extending the leg.

Safety and Alignment Tips

1. Maintain optimal body alignment as in the Back-of-Thigh Lift (move #42).

2. Avoid overstressing your knee. Make a right angle during bends, and be careful not to hyperextend the knee joint during extensions.

Stretch

Afterward, perform the Leg Hug (move #71).

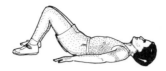

Move #44: The Buttocks Squeeze

How-To

While lying on your back with your knees bent, alternate contracting the muscles of your buttocks and then relaxing them.

Safety and Alignment Tips

1. To ensure mechanical efficiency, minimize any tendency to raise your hips high during squeezes. Your buttocks should lift only high enough to allow for a strong contraction. Concentrate on flexing your muscles, not on lifting your pelvis.
2. Do not hold contractions for more than a couple of seconds before relaxing.
3. Pay special attention to breathing naturally and regularly during this exercise.

Stretch

Afterward, perform the Leg Hug (move #71).

Frontal Thigh

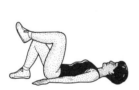 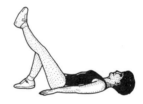

Move #45: Bend and Extend Forward

How-To

Alternate bending and extending the leg.

Safety and Alignment Tip

As with the Bend and Extend Backward exercise (move #43), avoid either overbending or hyperextending your knee joint.

Stretch

Afterward, perform the Gentle Quadriceps Stretch I (move #72).

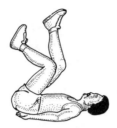

Move #46: The Bicycle

How-To

While lying on your back with your legs raised directly above the rest of your body, perform pedaling motions.

Safety and Alignment Tip

If you can do this comfortably, placing your hands beneath the buttocks can help to protect your back. For many mature exercisers, this position makes it easier to keep the lower spine flat on the floor and easier to hold the legs in *over* the body.

Stretch

Afterward, perform the Gentle Quadriceps Stretch II (move #73).

Inner Thighs

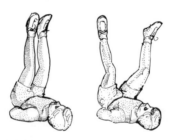

Move #47: In and Out at the Top

How-To

While lying on your back with your legs raised directly over the rest of your body, move your legs alternately together and then apart.

Safety and Alignment Tips

1. Separate your legs no more than approximately shoulder-width apart. It is unnecessary to perform a wider spread, which can, in fact, be hard on the hip joints.
2. As with the Bicycle (move #46), placing your hands beneath your buttocks can help to protect your back.
3. Keeping your knees slightly bent will reduce undue strain without diminishing the effectiveness of this exercise.

Stretch

Afterward, perform the Modified Straddle Stretch (move #74).

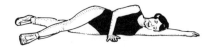

Move #48: The Inner Thigh Lift

How-To

While lying on your side, perform lifts with the lower leg.

Safety and Alignment Tips

1. Keep your spine optimally aligned by resting your head on your outstretched arm.
2. Relax your upper leg down to the front. By doing so, you will be able to position your upper hip directly over the lower one. Maintain this desirable hip-over-hip alignment by resting your foot on the floor and by relaxing your bent knee just above floor level.
3. The working leg's knee and toes should face the front, not the ceiling. The lifts should not be very high. Your working leg should be almost straight but short of locking the knee.

Stretch

Afterward, perform the Cross-Legged Stretch (move #75).

Outer Thighs

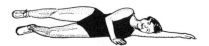

Move #49: The Outer Thigh Lift

How-To

While lying on your side, perform leg lifts with the upper leg.

Safety and Alignment Tips

1. As with the Inner Thigh Lift (move #48), ensure optimal spinal alignment by resting your head on your outstretched arm.
2. Relax the lower leg, bending it slightly.
3. Keep your upper hip directly above the lower hip. Do not permit your upper hip to roll backward.
4. The working leg's knee and toes should face the front, not the ceiling. Do not try to lift so high that your knee and toes tend to turn upward (you will wind up working the wrong muscle group!). The working leg should be almost straight but short of locking the knee. Perform all lifts directly above the anchored leg.

Stretch

Afterward, perform the Supine Outer Thigh Stretch (move #76).

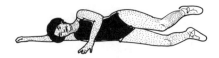

Move #50: The Bent Outer Thigh Lift

How-To

To make outer thigh work easier on the hip (or simply for vari-ety's sake), perform lifts with your knee bent.

Safety and Alignment Tip

Follow the alignment guidelines given for the Outer Thigh Lift (move #49).

Stretch

Afterward, perform the Seated Outer Thigh Stretch (move #77).

Shins and Calves

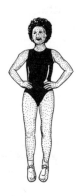

Move #51: Lift Onto Toes

How-To

Condition your calves by alternately raising your heels and then relaxing back down to the floor.

Safety and Alignment Tip

You may touch the wall or the back of a sturdy chair for balance during this exercise. When you grow sufficiently confident, per-form the exercise without touching, to promote your sense of balance.

Stretch

Afterward, perform the Wall Lower Leg Stretch (move #78).

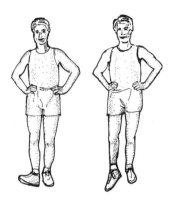

Move #52: The Flex/Point

How-To

Condition your calves and shins by alternately flexing the foot and then pointing the toes. Hold the foot that is flexing and pointing in front of you slightly above the floor.

Safety and Alignment Tip

Follow the balancing guidelines given for the Lift Onto Toes (move #51).

Variation

Flex-and-point movements may also be performed during leg lifts such as the Inner Thigh Lift (move #48) and the Outer Thigh Lift (move #49) in order to engage the calves and shins while working the primary muscles used for lifting.

Stretch

Afterward, perform the Floor Flex Stretch (move #79) and the Floor Point Stretch (move #81).

Feet and Toes

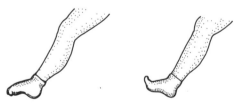

Move #53: Curl and Lift

How-To

Alternate curling your toes under and then raising them as high as possible.

Safety and Alignment Tip
This exercise can be done while lying on the floor, seated in a chair, or standing. Remember that the more stand-up exercises you perform, the more your skeletal system is likely to benefit. As with the Lift Onto Toes exercise (move #51), you may touch a stable object for balance or you can perform the exercise in a free-standing position to promote your sense of balance.

Stretch
Afterward, perform the Kneeling Stretch (move #80).

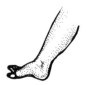

Move #54: Wriggling

How-To
Wriggle the toes pleasurably for about 30 seconds to 1 minute.

Safety and Alignment Tip
Refer to the instructions accompanying the Curl and Lift (move #53) for the various positions in which this exercise may be performed.

Stretch
Afterward, perform the Kneeling Stretch (move #80).

CHAPTER 6

Stretch Exercise So Joints Don't Get Set in Their Ways

The term *range of motion* means the flexibility of a joint. As we grow older, the tissues around our joints tend to thicken and lose pliability. Muscles may grow shorter. Range of motion decreases. Stretch exercise combats these tendencies, thereby helping us to remain active and self-sufficient.

TYPES OF STRETCH EXERCISES

Some of the most supple people in the world are ballet dancers. Even so, dance is well known for sacrificing physiological principle in favor of aesthetic achievement. Because certain ballet exercises involve extreme and unusual stretches of the limbs, the mature adult is cautioned that this art may lead to injury, particularly of the knees. The same is true of yoga. However, gentle ballet and yoga programs especially developed for the adult are available in some areas. These programs do not include questionable or high-risk stretches.

Swimming and water activities in general are excellent for increasing flexibility. Many adults enjoy a wider range of motion in water, thanks to a reduction of gravitational pull. This decrease in gravity reduces pressure effects on the joints, freeing them to better perform desired movements.

For overall flexibility, a conservative basic stretch program is hard to beat. Such a program is provided in this chapter.

HOW HARD, HOW LONG, HOW OFTEN

There should be nothing hard about your stretch exercise program. This is a time to relax and enjoy! Each stretch should be pursued to a degree at which your muscle feels stretched but not distressed. Stretches should be conservative, so that no muscle ever feels more than just *slightly* uncomfortable, if that. Never force any stretch. Never try to stretch so far that you experience pain.

Taking your time, ease into each separate stretch. Hold the stretch for 15 to 30 seconds. Perform the stretch three times, taking a moment to rest between repetitions. Move on to the next stretch and repeat the procedure. Remember to breathe naturally and regularly during each stretch.

To preserve your current level of flexibility, perform your stretch routine three times a week, spaced out over the course of each week. To increase flexibility, stretch 4 or 5 days per week.

As you progress, increasing the challenge of your flexibility program is easy. Just stretch farther as you find that you are naturally able to do so without encountering pain. You may also vary or add new stretches to your routine.

STRETCHING FOR SPECIAL CONDITIONS

Although people with asthma may have difficulty obtaining medical approval for aerobic exercise (due to the very real potential for complications upon strenuous exertion), most physicians recognize the value of gentle stretch exercise in coping with the condition.

A doctor may prescribe medications such as bronchodilators, which serve to widen the air passages by relaxing smooth bronchial muscle. Such medications may allow people with asthma to exercise more freely.

Stretch is a key element in the prevention and treatment of lower back pain. For starters, increasing flexibility promotes better posture. Poor posture contributes to back pain by promoting misalignment of the spine. Tightness in the muscles of the back and upper legs produces additional back pain by increasing curvature of the spine.

To discourage back problems, pay particular attention to stretches for the hamstrings (back of thigh), the abdomen, the buttocks, and for the back and shoulder girdle area. But do not neglect other muscles. A program aimed at limbering the entire body will be most beneficial. All of the stretches included in the Full Life exercise selection are especially designed to help prevent undue stress to the back. Aging connective tissue and support muscles may not provide adequate control with regard to gravity and body weight when the spine is stretched into a swayback position during standing exercise. Therefore, no Full Life exercises suggest that type of stretch. Usually, arched extension can be performed safely on the floor from a prone position while the body is supported by both hands (with the elbow joints unlocked). However, the Full Life exercise selection does not include that stretch, because many adults already tend to sway the back during everyday activities or as the result of postural flaws.

Stretch exercise can be very important in the management of arthritis. Because the structures of joint and muscle tissue are elastic, steps should be taken to prevent them from growing tighter and more restricted. In this way, stretch exercise can help to preserve the declining range of motion.

Gentleness is a special must in stretch programs for people with back problems, arthritis, osteoporosis, or any condition likely to decrease the natural range of motion. Physical limitations must be respected. Stretches never should be forced but should, instead, be pursued to a degree that fully employs the existing range. With practice and patience, that range gradually will broaden. For people with reduced flexibility, it may be practical to use towels or other assistive devices during stretch exercise sessions. Overweight individuals—as well as people with hypertension or diabetes—stand to gain the same general benefits that other exercisers enjoy through range of motion endeavors. People with *any* type of medical disorder should consult with their physicians about performing physical exercise, including stretch activity.

Many adults find stretch exercise to be a singularly relaxing and pleasurable pastime. For this reason, it is high on the list as an effective stress management tool.

FULL LIFE STRETCH EXERCISE PROGRAM

The Full Life stretch plan has been carefully developed to provide the mature adult with all the benefits of stretch exercise while minimizing risk of injury. Note that the exercise selection does not include controversial stretches or positions known to be risky. This plan excludes the "hurdler's stretch," which strains the knee severely. It excludes the "plow," which places far too much pressure on the neck. Nor will you be asked to attempt radical stretches that contort the spine or twist the limbs.

Instead, you will master pure-and-simple stretches that complement the natural structure of your body. So, instead of forcing your body to attempt unnatural feats, you will improve its ability to function as it was made to do! Table 6.1 offers a practical format for stretching.

TABLE 6.1

Practical Format for a Stretch Workout
• General warm-up—10 to 15 minutes • Stretches—30 to 40 minutes   Choose one or two exercises for each body region.

Additionally, the Full Life stretch plan addresses areas of special concern to mature adults. For example, it is important to pay attention to your chest muscles over the years, for when those muscles grow short from disuse, respiration may be hampered. One prevalent cause of disability in later life is a shortening of the

Achilles tendon. And once that tendon forfeits flexibility, it is very difficult to restore. Therefore, its preservation is a built-in feature of the Full Life stretch plan.

Here are essential rules to follow for safe and successful stretching:

- Although all of the following exercises involve assuming only the gentlest and most natural positions, some people's bodies still aren't made to perform certain stretches comfortably. If any stretch hurts or feels abnormal to you, omit it from your regimen.
- Never bounce during any stretch. Instead, ease into the stretched position and hold it in a relaxed manner.
- During flexibility work, you may fully extend a stretching limb. As with other forms of exercise, however, you should avoid *hyperextending* any joint. In other words, do not overdo it by forcing your joint to overstretch beyond its natural range of motion. This rule applies to *all* exercises, including *all* of the following stretches. Your Full Life stretch exercise instructions provide reminders to avoid hyperextension and point out specific stretches that most often "tempt" exercisers to overdo.
- Remember *never* to hold your breath. Always breathe naturally and regularly during your stretch workout.
- Before stretching, perform a thorough warm-up as described in chapter 3. No cool-down period is required after stretching. In fact, your stretch routine serves well as the final activity after aerobic or calisthenic workouts.
- Perform at least one stretch for each body section.

As with other forms of exercise, the use of music during stretch exercise is optional, but unlike other forms of exercise, stretching should not be performed *to the beat of* musical accompaniment. Instead, slow and relaxing tunes should be played gently in the background to create an atmosphere of tranquility and peacefulness. Choose beautiful music that encourages a sense of quiet harmony. Never hurry, just slow down and enjoy. Stretch smoothly; breathe luxuriously; relax completely.

Stretch Exercises

The Neck

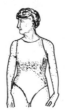

Move #55: The Head Turn

How-To

Gently and slowly turn your head to look to one side. Hold for a few moments before turning to look to the other side.

Safety and Alignment Tips

1. Movements involving the neck should always be performed cautiously and conservatively.
2. Neck movements may be performed while seated on the floor, seated in a chair, or standing. Standing best promotes skeletal health. Mature adults are advised not to close their eyes while standing, because one's sense of balance grows more dependent upon vision as one gets older. Maintain optimal stand-up posture as described in chapter 3. Or if you choose a seated position, remember never to slump but to sit up straight instead.

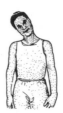

Move #56: The Head Tilt

How-To

Gently and slowly tilt one ear toward your shoulder. Hold for a few moments before tilting the other ear toward your opposite shoulder.

Safety and Alignment Tips

1. It is not necessary for the mature adult to place a hand on the head, pulling or pressing the head in one direction or another. That practice could prove detrimental by overstretching the

tissues of the neck. Remember that all movements involving the neck should be performed cautiously and conservatively.

2. Refer to instructions for the Head Turn (move #55) for safety information regarding the various positions in which this exercise may be performed.

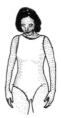

Move #57: The Nod

How-To

Gently and slowly nod toward the front, hold for a few moments, and then return your head to a natural, erect position.

Safety and Alignment Tips

1. When you lift your head, raise it to a level at which you are looking straight ahead, not up toward the ceiling. Tilting the head backward places unnecessary strain on the vertebrae of your neck. Likewise shun head rolls, because they produce the same effect. Remember that all movements involving the neck should be performed cautiously and conservatively.

2. Refer to instructions for the Head Turn (move #55) for safety information regarding the various positions in which this exercise may be performed.

Shoulder Region and Triceps

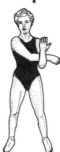

Move #58: The Stretch-Across

How-To

1. Stretch one arm across your chest. Place it in the bend of your opposite elbow.

2. You may increase the stretch by gently pressing upward and backward with the bent arm.

Safety and Alignment Tip

Do this exercise standing, if you can, to promote skeletal health, and maintain optimal stand-up posture as described in chapter 3. If you choose to do this stretch while seated in a chair or on the floor, remember never to slump or slouch. Think of yourself as "sitting tall in the saddle."

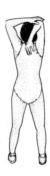

Move #59: The Big Stretch

How-To

Place hand #1 at the back of your neck. Grasp its elbow with hand #2, and pull it slowly and gently toward the back of the head. Repeat with the other arm.

Safety and Alignment Tip

Regarding posture, see the safety information for the Stretch-Across (move #58).

Variation

If this stretch is difficult for you, stick with the Stretch-Across (move #58). All in good time, you may find that you can successfully perform this stretch also.

Shoulder Region and Biceps

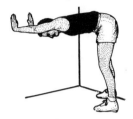

Move #60: The Wall Stretch

How-To

With both palms against a wall to support your spine, bend from the hips until the top of your head points toward the wall.

Safety and Alignment Tip

Be careful not to hyperextend your elbows, not to lock your knees, not to go swayback, and not to crane your neck or "droop" your head downward. Instead, make an effort to line up the vertebrae of your neck with those in the rest of your spine.

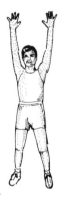

Move #61: The Upward Reach

How-To

Stretch both arms up luxuriously.

Safety and Alignment Tip

Regarding posture, see the safety information for the Stretch-Across (move #58).

Variation

If you have trouble reaching overhead, then stretch your arms forward at chest level or outward at shoulder level.

Forearms, Wrists, and Fingers

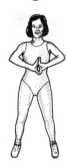

Move #62: The Steepling Stretch

How-To

With fingers pointing inward, match the fingertips of one hand with those of the other.

Safety and Alignment Tips

1. Do not push the hands together in a strained fashion. Instead, simply touch in order to enjoy a pleasant stretch throughout the hands, fingers, and wrists.
2. Regarding posture, see the safety information for the Stretch-Across (move #58).

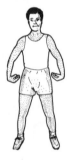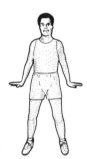

Move #63: Turning the Hands

How-To

Turn your hands inward and upward as high as is comfortable. After holding this position for a few moments, lift your hands as high as is comfortable in the opposite direction. Hold for a few moments before relaxing your hands into their natural position.

Safety and Alignment Tip

Regarding posture, see the safety information for the Stretch-Across (move #58).

Variation

You may also turn your hands toward each side in the manner described here.

Chest

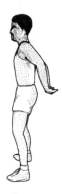

Move #64: The Chest Stretcher

How-To

Holding your hands together behind your back, stretch your arms backward and upward.

Safety and Alignment Tip

Pay particular attention to keeping your elbows and knees relaxed and your back straight, not swayback.

Variation

If you have trouble holding your hands together, simply stretch your arms backward and upward.

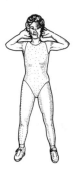

Move #65: The Bent Stretch

How-To

With your fingertips touching your head behind your ears, gently direct your elbows backward.

Safety and Alignment Tip
Regarding posture, see the safety information for the Stretch-Across (move #58).

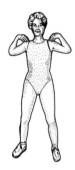

Move #66: The Shoulder-Touch Stretch

How-To
With your fingertips touching the top of your shoulders, gently direct your elbows backward.

Safety and Alignment Tip
Regarding posture, see the safety information for the Stretch-Across (move #58).

Midsection

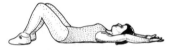

Move #67: The Midsection Stretch

How-To
With your knees bent, reach both arms overhead.

Safety and Alignment Tips
1. Your arms may rest on the floor as you stretch. Remember to keep your stretch gentle by avoiding any tendency to hyperextend the elbow joints.
2. Be sure to keep your lower back securely on the floor.

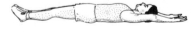

Move #68: The Full Body Stretch

How-To
Stretch your arms in one direction and your legs in the other.

Safety and Alignment Tip

Your limbs may rest on the floor as you stretch. Avoid any tendency to hyperextend the elbow or knee joints as you stretch.

Variation

Most mature adults can perform this stretch successfully, and in fact, many find it to be particularly relaxing and pleasurable. However, if you cannot keep your lower back from arching stressfully upward from the floor during this stretch, then stick with the Midsection Stretch (move #67).

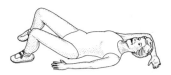

Move #69: The One-Side-at-a-Time Stretch

How-To

With your knees bent, relax one arm down by your side and bend the other arm above your head. After holding that attitude for a few moments, reverse arm positions.

Safety and Alignment Tip

As in the Midsection Stretch (move #67) and the Full Body Stretch (move #68), pay special attention to keeping your lower back securely on the floor.

Back, Buttocks, and Hamstrings

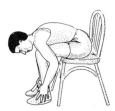

Move #70: The Chair Stretch

How-To

Slowly allow your upper body to bend forward from the hips as far as feels natural and comfortable.

Safety and Alignment Tip

To make certain that your spine is properly supported at all times during this stretch, walk or slide your hands down your legs as you lower your body. As you relax into your stretch, rest your torso on your upper legs and place both hands on your ankles. As you rise, walk or slide your hands up your legs.

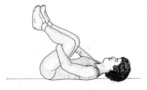

Move #71: The Leg Hug

How-To
While lying on your back, pull your legs very gently in toward your chest.

Safety and Alignment Tip
Be sure to place your hands on your thighs behind your knees rather than around your knees. This technique eliminates undue strain on the knee joints.

Frontal Thighs

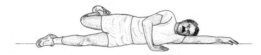

Move #72: The Gentle Quadriceps Stretch I

How-To
Lie on your side with your head resting on your outstretched arm, your upper hip positioned directly above the lower hip, and your lower knee relaxed. Gently bend the upper knee until you feel a pleasant stretch at the front of your thigh.

Safety and Alignment Tips
1. You need not perform a severe knee bend to elongate the quadriceps. If you feel a pulling sensation in or around your knee, you are bending too far—decrease the degree of your bend.
2. It is not necessary to reach behind with your upper arm and pull the leg into a bend. In many mature adults, doing so will result in a bend that is too harsh on the knee joint. Employ that technique only if you can do so with relative ease, without a pulling sensation at the knee, and if you feel that it helps your leg to relax into the stretch.

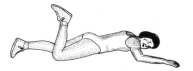

Move #73: The Gentle Quadriceps Stretch II

How-To

Lying prone with your neck and shoulders in a nonstressful position, gently bend your leg upward from the knee until you feel a pleasant stretch at the front of your thigh.

Safety and Alignment Tip

Observe the special safety precautions given for the Gentle Quadriceps Stretch I (move #72).

Inner Thighs

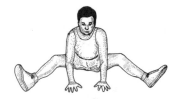

Move #74: The Modified Straddle Stretch

How-To

With your knees bent and your legs separated only as far as feels comfortable, place both hands on the floor to support your back as you relax the upper body forward. This will stretch several parts of your body.

Safety and Alignment Tips

1. Be sure to keep your elbows relaxed during this stretch.
2. Do not worry if you cannot stretch very far toward the front during this stretch. Simply relax forward as far as feels natural. It is a good idea to think in terms of stretching *forward* rather than *downward*.

Move #75: The Cross-Legged Stretch

How-To

Assume a cross-legged position being careful not to overbend your knees. Keeping both hands on the floor at all times, ease your upper body forward. This will stretch several parts of your body.

Safety and Alignment Tips

1. Support your back by walking your hands forward on the floor as you bend and then by walking them in again as you rise. Remember to keep your elbows unlocked throughout the process.
2. Regarding the degree of your stretch, follow the safety guidelines given for the Modified Straddle Stretch (move #74).

Outer Thighs

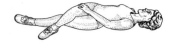

Move #76: The Supine Outer Thigh Stretch

How-To

Lying on your back, bend one leg and cross it over the other. With your opposite hand, gently press your knee toward the floor.

Safety and Alignment Tip

In holding your leg with your hand, do not press so hard that you feel any pulling sensation. Instead, keep your press conservative, drawing the knee gently downward until you feel a pleasant stretch in the outer thigh region.

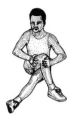

Move #77: The Seated Outer Thigh Stretch

How-To

In a seated position, bend one leg across the other, supporting the bent knee with both hands. Gently press your knee inward toward your chest.

Safety and Alignment Tips

1. Don't slump! Maintain good seated posture.
2. Be sure to relax the knee of your extended leg.
3. As with the Supine Outer Thigh Stretch (move #76), do not press so hard with your hands that you feel any pulling sensation. Instead, keep the press conservative, drawing the knee gently inward until a pleasant stretch is achieved.

Calves, Achilles Tendons, and Ankles

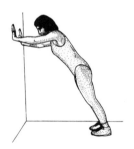

Move #78: The Wall Lower Leg Stretch

How-To

With both hands on the wall, lean forward, keeping your heels on the floor.

Safety and Alignment Tip

Remember to keep your back straight (not swayback) and to relax your knees and elbows.

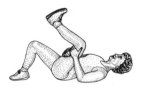

Move #79: The Floor Flex Stretch

How-To

Lying on your back with one leg bent, hold the other leg by placing both hands behind the knee. Flex the foot, drawing your toes toward the front of your leg.

Safety and Alignment Tip

When you perform this stretch, be sure to place your hands behind the knee (on your thigh), not around it.

Shins, Ankles, and Feet

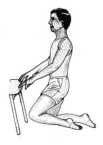

Move #80: The Kneeling Stretch

How-To

Supported by a sturdy chair, kneel on the floor. Lift one knee and move it slightly forward. Gently press the top of your foot to the floor.

Variation

You may wish to place a thin pillow or a folded towel beneath your knees during this stretch.

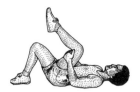

Move #81: The Floor Point Stretch

How-To

Lying on your back with one leg bent, hold the other leg by placing both hands behind the knee. Point your toes.

Safety and Alignment Tip

When you perform this stretch, be sure to place your hands behind the knee (on your thigh), not around it.

CHAPTER 7

Water Workouts for Staying in the Swim

Whether you are an experienced exerciser or a novice, water exercise may be just the ticket for increasing the pleasure and benefits gained through your physical fitness program. Pool exercise offers the regular exerciser an enjoyable option for cross-training—that is, changing your regimen occasionally so you won't feel like you're stuck in a rut. For the sedentary individual, water work provides an easy-does-it approach to renewed physical activity.

You need not be a swimmer to enjoy pool workouts, because the exercises are designed to be performed in shallow water.

HOW HARD, HOW LONG, HOW OFTEN

For calisthenic work, pool exercise principles are similar to those for land exercise. The biggest difference is that water must be displaced by your body to accomplish calisthenic movements in a swimming pool. Therefore, the water itself provides considerable resistance, which is a plus for your muscular system. Each exercise should be continued until the working muscle feels fatigued. Mature adults should then stretch the area for 10 to 15 seconds before proceeding to the next calisthenic exercise. Ideally, calisthenics should be performed three times spaced out over the course of each week. The workouts could be all water work, all land work, or a combination such as 2 days of work on land and 1 day in the water. To increase the challenge as you grow stronger, add repetitions, master new water exercises, and perform arm motions with your hands cupped rather than with your fingers spread apart. Or try wearing fins during leg exercises and holding fins during work involving your arms. Observe all of the special safety guidelines given for calisthenic exercise in chapter 5.

As with land exercise, water stretches undertaken to enhance flexibility should be held for 15 to 30 seconds and performed three times apiece. Stretch exercise should be performed 3 to 5 days per week, depending upon whether you are simply trying to maintain your present level of flexibility or whether your aim is to increase range of motion. As with calisthenics, it is fine to combine stretch sessions in the pool with sessions performed on land to add variety and pleasure to your overall fitness program. The range and depth of your stretches should increase gradually as you grow more flexible. Observe all of the special safety guidelines given for stretch exercise in chapter 6.

When it comes to aerobics, there is a modification suggested for mature adults moving from the land into the water. Reduce your training heart rate goal by 5 to 10 beats per minute for water aerobics. For example, if your training rate goal is 110 beats per minute on land, aim for 105 or 100 in the water. The aerobic session should last from 20 to 30 minutes and should be performed at least three times spaced out over the course of each week. Observe all of the special guidelines given for aerobic exercise in chapter 4.

As with calisthenics and stretch, it is perfectly fine to please yourself in structuring your aerobic exercise agenda. You can perform all of the aerobic exercise you need in the pool or all on land. You can alternate 1 week in the pool and then the next week on land. Or you might opt for one aerobic session on land and two in the pool over the course of any given week. To increase the challenge, lengthen your workout, perform more energetically, or introduce new aerobic patterns and combinations into your pool routine.

POOL WORK FOR SPECIAL CONDITIONS

Pool exercise is widely appreciated by people with arthritis. Indeed, when pain is a significant factor, water work may be the only practical form of physical exercise. While submerged in water, your body weighs only 10% of its weight on land. For this reason, water exercise is kinder to joints, bones, tendons, ligaments, and muscles than most land exercise. Due to the reduction of gravitational pull, a wider range of motion is enjoyed in water—a feature of pool exercise that promotes *success* for the arthritis sufferer. Whereas a water temperature of from 78 to 84 degrees Fahrenheit is recommended for the general population, the warmer end of that range is preferable for people with arthritis. Additionally, people with arthritis should perform only low-impact aerobic movements, whether on land or in the water.

For all of these reasons, water workouts are also especially beneficial for people with back problems, knee or hip weakness, osteoporosis, or any other disorder that limits musculoskeletal strength. Working out in water effectively banishes fears of falling.

As with other forms of exercise, it is imperative that people with *any* types of medical disorders cooperate fully with their physicians in performing swimming pool activity. With medical approval, people with conditions ranging from asthma to diabetes and hypertension may enjoy the advantages of water exercise.

The buoyancy provided by water takes most of the jolt out of exercise. Therefore, many people who could never safely run, hop, or kick on land can do so viably while supported by water. However, all mature exercisers are cautioned to monitor the response of joint tissue to movements that involve bouncing or jumping—*even in water*. If your joints feel stressed or you experience pain, eliminate bouncy moves from your workout and stick with the low-impact alternative exercises described in the aerobic workout section of this chapter.

Performing water aerobics is an excellent way to promote weight loss. When the body is heavy, joints must bear an extreme load during weight-bearing activity on land. But this pressure is diminished in the water. Additionally, there is no reason to feel self-conscious about displaying an imperfect figure when working in waist-high or chest-high water.

Water exercise is especially effective for the reduction of normal, everyday stress. The smooth, fluid quality of a water workout tends to relieve tension and to increase one's sense of well-being. As you exercise in a pool, water actually massages your body, producing a soothing effect both physically and emotionally.

WARMING UP AND COOLING DOWN

For the first 6 or 7 minutes of a water workout, walk in the pool at an easy pace or perform very light, slow versions of the aerobic movements described in this chapter (or do both). Follow this by giving your body a 5- or 6-minute leisurely preview of the muscle and joint work to come later in your pool workout. Warm-up work should always be performed at a low intensity level. Special attention should be paid to limbering up your back. In group situations, it is fun to top off the warm-up period by tossing a beach ball from person to person.

For an alternative pool warm-up, stand on the pool deck and follow the warm-up instructions for land-based workouts given in chapter 3. Shoes should be worn during this type of warm-up.

Perform a thorough warm-up whether you intend to perform an aerobic, calisthenic, stretch, or total-body workout. See Table 7.1.

To cool down after pool aerobics, walk or dance lightly for 6 or 7 minutes as previously described. Continue this activity until your pulse rate descends below 100 beats per minute. If it remains above 100 beats per minute, perform gentler movements until your pulse rate descends. Then enjoy the swimming pool stretch routine given in this chapter. To cool down after pool calisthenics, perform the stretch routine.

If you want to accomplish a total-body workout during one pool exercise session, first perform the aforementioned warm-up. Complete your aerobic work. Then perform a mildly active, standing cool-down for 6 to 7 minutes. Continue this activity until your pulse rate descends below 100 beats per minute. If it remains over 100 beats per minute, perform gentler movements until your pulse rate

TABLE 7.1

Practical Format for a Water Workout Warm-Up

- **Limber up—6 to 7 minutes**
    Good limbering movements include easy-paced versions of the following movements: walking, marching in place, the Shift (move #82), the low-impact variation for the Modified Leg-Out Jumping Jack (move #89), the low-impact variation for Kicking (move #90—with low arm reaches, too, if that feels more comfortable as you begin your workout), and the low-impact variation for Bobbing (move #91).

- **Rhythmical exercise—5 to 6 minutes**
    Good rhythmical warm-ups include brief and relaxed, nonstrenuous versions of the following movements: the Shift (move #82), the Standing Swim (move #92—try this with fingers separated during the warm-up and then with hands cupped later during the calisthenic segment of the workout), the Standing Scissor (move #96), the Pool Cat Curl (move #97), the Doorknob (move #99), the Quadriceps Firmer (move #110), and the Figure Eight With Foot (move #113).

- **Very mild stretching—1 to 2 minutes**
    Good warm-up stretches include very conservative versions of the following movements: the Good Posture Stretch (move #115), Reaching for the Sky (move #117), the Elbows Backward Stretch (move #121), the Wet Leg-Hug Stretch (move #124), the Wet Point Stretch (move #128), and the Wet Flex Stretch (move #129).

descends. Stretch your calves and hamstrings, and then complete your calisthenics routine. End with the stretch routine. See Table 7.2.

FULL LIFE WATER WORKOUT PROGRAM

This chapter provides instructions for three types of pool workouts: (a) aerobics, (b) calisthenics, and (c) stretch. Follow the warm-up

TABLE 7.2

Practical Format for a Water-Based Cool-Down After Aerobics
• **Standing cool-down—5 to 7 minutes (longer if needed for heart rate recovery)** Good standing cool-down activities include easy-paced versions of the following movements: walking, marching in place, the Shift (move #82), the low-impact variation for the Modified Leg-Out Jumping Jack (move #89), the low-impact variation for Kicking (move #90—with low arm reaches, too, during your cool-down), and the low-impact variation for Bobbing (move #91).
• **If you plan to perform muscle-conditioning activities in the same workout, you should take a moment to stretch your calves and hamstrings before proceeding to your calisthenic exercises and then to your final cool-down stretches.** Use the Wet Leg-Hug Stretch (move #124) and the Wet Flex Stretch (move #129).
• **Stretches—5 minutes (or more)** Perform the swimming pool stretch routine (moves #115 through #129).

and cool-down directions given in the preceding section before and after pool exercise.

The aerobic exercises should be performed in water at *least* waist high, to prevent excessive impact.

Remember that the cooling quality of the water will lessen your awareness of heat and perspiration. Do keep a nonbreakable container of water handy to replenish lost fluids during your water workout.

Always wear an effective sunscreen for all outdoor activity, including work in the pool.

As in all Full Life exercises, you should avoid joint hyperextension (as defined in chapter 3) throughout swimming pool work. When you are standing in water, maintain optimal posture as described in chapter 3. Instructions for many of the water exercises include special reminders regarding good alignment and proper exercise methods. These additional reminders accompany certain moves during which some exercisers tend to forget the rules for model posture and optimal technique.

Music can add to the beauty and pleasure of water exercise. Be careful, however, never to touch electronic sound equipment (or anything else electric) when you are wet or standing on a damp surface. If you want your aerobic and calisthenic activities to match the beat of your musical selections, keep in mind that water reduces speed of movement. So select tunes with a slower tempo than those used for land exercise. Do not try to perform your stretch routine in compliance with any musical beat; instead, choose slow and flowing music to lend a feeling of serenity to your stretch exercise atmosphere. If you like, you can perform your entire pool workout without trying to coordinate your exercise movements with the rhythms of musical numbers. For example, you might perform warm-up, aerobic, calisthenic, and stretch work while inspirational symphony music plays softly in the background.

As previously mentioned, the mature exerciser should stretch a muscle or muscle group once for 10 to 15 seconds after engaging it in calisthenic exercise. After doing so, you are ready to begin the next calisthenic activity. Each muscular conditioning exercise for the pool is accompanied by the name and number of an appropriate stretch for this purpose.

When doing swimming pool exercises, observe all of the good-sense safety guidelines discussed in chapter 3. As with all components of the Full Life Fitness program, water exercise should be approached with an attitude of moderation. Instead of "going for the burn," go for the fun! Unlike the land workouts presented in previous chapters, the following pool workouts do not include a selection of exercises for every major muscle group. So instead of choosing at least one exercise for each body section, try to perform *every* exercise given in the following workouts. Remember, you can perform aerobics-only, calisthenics-only, stretch-only, or total-body workouts. To avoid overexertion, follow the instructions provided in this chapter under the heading "How Hard, How Long, How Often." If any specific movement feels unpleasant or painful to you, then strike it from your personal exercise plan.

Now that we have explored the principles of water exercise, let's get wet!

Swimming Pool Exercises

Aerobics

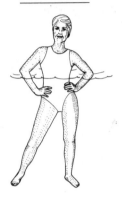

Move #82: The Shift

How-To

1. Shift your hips from side to side.
2. This movement is a low-intensity exercise. Use it to "get your-self going," to pace yourself when you feel the need to light-en up, and to slow things down toward the end of your aerobic session.

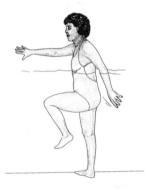

Move #83: Walking

How-To

Walk briskly back and forth across the shallow end of the pool. Swing your arms at your sides as you walk. Make several round-trips.

Variations

1. Try making one round-trip walking lightly on your heels.
2. Try a round-trip walking lightly on your toes.
3. Try walking sideways.

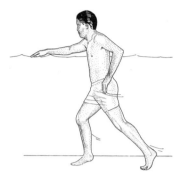

Move #84: Jogging
How-To

Jog lightly back and forth across the shallow end of the pool. The resistance of the water limits speed, so take long, leaping steps and use your arms to help pull your body through the water. Make several round-trips.

Variations
1. If leap-jogging feels too strenuous for your joints, substitute walking, with an emphasis on taking big steps to achieve a long stride.
2. For added challenge, try Walking (move #83) and Jogging (move #84) in relatively deep (chest-high) water.
3. Optional: Swim one or two laps across the shallow end of your pool.

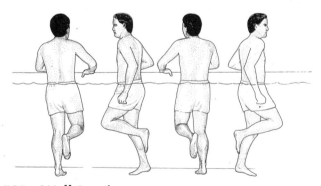

Move #85: Wall Jogging
How-To

Face the side wall of the pool. Touch your hands to the wall for balance, and jog lightly in place. Concentrate on keeping your leg movements energetic. After about a minute, turn your right side to the wall. Keeping your right hand on the wall for balance, continue jogging in place energetically. After another minute, repeat while facing the wall again. Then repeat with your left side to the wall.

Variations

1. You can also jog in place while free-standing in the center of the shallow end of the pool. For variety, turn occasionally as you jog.
2. If jogging in place feels too strenuous for your joints, substitute walking in place, with an emphasis on taking very quick steps while free-standing or while touching the pool wall as pictured.

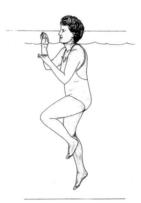

Move #86: Treading Water

How-To

1. Using all four limbs, tread water for about 3 minutes in neck-high water.
2. Do not overexert. Because you are in shallow water, simply touch the floor with your toes occasionally as necessary. Your goal is to need fewer and fewer floor touches.

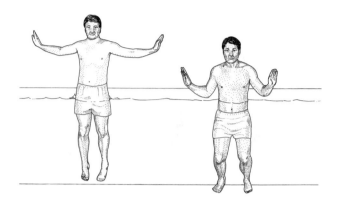

Move #87: Hopping

How-To

Hop lightly on both feet while pushing both arms out to your sides above the water.

Safety and Alignment Tip

Remember never to lock your knees upon landing.

Variation

If hopping feels too strenuous for your joints, substitute shifting or walking in place while performing the arm movements pictured.

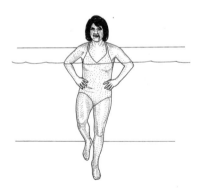

Move #88: The Alternate Hop

How-To

With hands on hips, alternate hopping lightly on your right foot two times and hopping on your left foot two times.

Safety and Alignment Tip

Never lock your knee upon landing.

Variations

1. For variety, alternate hopping four times per foot. For joint safety, do not exceed that number.

2. If hopping feels too strenuous for your joints, substitute marching in place while swinging your arms actively through the water at your sides.

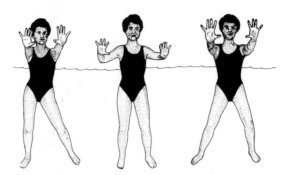

Move #89: The Modified Leg-Out Jumping Jack

How-To

Spring upward, clearing both feet off the floor, as you extend your right leg out to touch down lightly at the side upon descent. Then spring upward as you bring your legs together to touch down lightly at the center. Repeat, extending the left leg. Push both arms to the front above the water's surface as your legs extend. Continue alternating.

Safety and Alignment Tip

Never lock your knees upon landing.

Variation

If jumping feels too strenuous for your joints, perform this exercise without springing. Keeping at least one foot in contact with the floor at all times, simply alternately extend one leg and then the other while performing the arm movements pictured.

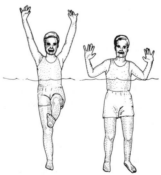

Move #90: Kicking

How-To

Perform "chorus line" kicks while pushing both arms high overhead.

Safety and Alignment Tips
1. Don't try to kick *too* high. That can be hard on your hips.
2. Never lock your knees upon landing.

Variations
1. If it is difficult for you to reach high overhead, then simply reach to a height that feels comfortable.
2. If kicking feels too strenuous for your joints, perform this exercise without jumping upward as you kick. Keeping at least one foot in contact with the floor at all times, alternately lift one leg and then the other energetically while performing the arm movements pictured.

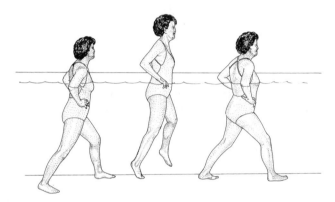

Move #91: Bobbing

How-To
Extend your right leg rearward while your left knee remains bent at the front, and then quickly reverse leg positions. Continue alternating.

Safety and Alignment Tips
1. Your front knee should always remain *behind* your front toes. Otherwise, you may needlessly tax your leg by overbending it.
2. Remember not to lock either leg upon landing.

Variation
This action requires lifting both feet clear of the pool bottom simultaneously. If that feels too strenuous for your joints, substitute a low-impact version. Keeping at least one foot in contact with the pool bottom at all times, simply extend your right leg rearward and then return it so that you are again standing with both feet side by side. Repeat with the left leg, and continue alternating.

Calisthenics

Upper Body

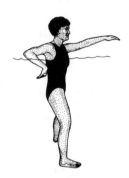

Move #92: The Standing Swim

How-To

Reach toward the front with one hand. Pull downward through the water, drawing your hand back to your thigh. Repeat with the other hand, and continue alternating as though you were swimming.

Variation

If possible, cup your hands for added resistance. If a less strenuous version is needed, separate your fingers.

Stretch

Afterward, perform Reaching for the Sky (move #117).

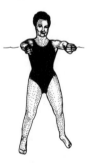

Move #93: The Standing Breast Stroke

How-To

With your arms submerged, use your arms and shoulders to imitate the swimming breast stroke. Palms face outward.

Variation

Increase or decrease resistance as outlined in the Standing Swim (move #92).

Stretch

Afterward, perform Reaching for the Sky (move #117).

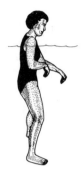

Move #94: The Standing Dog Paddle

How-To

With your arms submerged, use your arms and shoulders to imitate the dog-paddle stroke.

Variation

Increase or decrease resistance as outlined in the Standing Swim (move #92).

Stretch

Afterward, perform Reaching for the Sky (move #117).

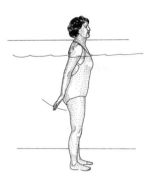

Move #95: The Rearward Push

How-To

Begin with both arms down by your sides, palms facing backward. Perform arm lifts toward the back.

Safety and Alignment Tip

Be especially careful not to lock your elbows during this exercise.

Variation

Increase or decrease resistance as outlined in the Standing Swim (move #92).

Stretch

Afterward, perform the Elbows Up Stretch (move #120).

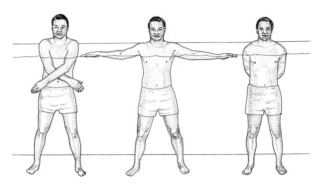

Move #96: The Standing Scissor

How-To

Cross your arms in front of your body, open out to the sides, and then cross behind your back. Continue alternating.

Safety and Alignment Tip

Pay particular attention to keeping your knees relaxed and your back straight during this exercise.

Stretch

Afterward, perform the Elbows Up Stretch (move #120).

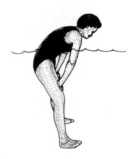

Move #97: The Pool Cat Curl

How-To

Perform the Standing Cat Curl (move #29) in waist- to chest-high water.

Safety and Alignment Tip

Be sure to follow the safety guidelines given with the Standing Cat Curl (move #29).

Stretch

Afterward, perform the Wet Leg-Hug Stretch (move #124).

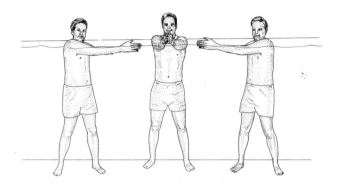

Move #98: Turning

How-To
Begin with both arms in front of your chest at the water's surface. Your arms should be close together with palms touching. Gently pull your arms toward one side and then toward the other side.

Safety and Alignment Tip
Keep your movements smooth, deliberate, and moderately slow to prevent jerking your spine or twisting it excessively.

Stretch
Afterward, perform Reaching for the Sky (move #117).

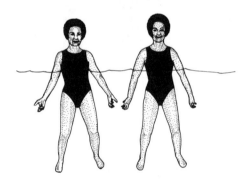

Move #99: The Doorknob

How-To
With your arms submerged, turn your hands back and forth as though you were turning a doorknob.

Stretch
Afterward, perform Bending at the Wrists (move #119).

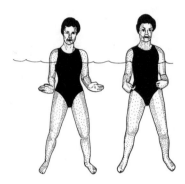

Move #100: The Wrist Worker

How-To

With your arms submerged, cup your hands. Alternate bending your hands back toward the tops of your wrists and then in toward the insides of your wrists.

Stretch

Afterward, perform Bending at the Wrists (move #119).

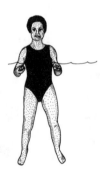

Move #101: The Pool Open and Close

How-To

Perform the Open and Close (move #27) with your hands submerged.

Safety and Alignment Tip

Be sure to follow the safety guidelines for the Open and Close (move #27).

Stretch

Afterward, perform the Feel-Good Stretch (move #118).

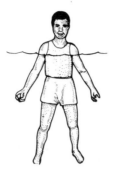

Move #102: The Pool Thumb to Fingertips

How-To

Perform the Thumb to Fingertips (move #26) with your hands submerged.

Stretch

Afterward, perform the Feel-Good Stretch (move #118).

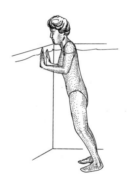

Move #103: The Pool Push-Up

How-To

Perform Wall Push-Ups (move #33), using your pool wall.

Safety and Alignment Tip

Be sure to follow the safety guidelines for Wall Push-Ups (move #33).

Stretch

Afterward, perform the Elbows Backward Stretch (move #121).

Midsection

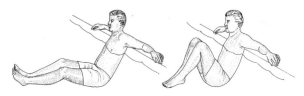

Move #104: The Pool Wall Knee Lift

How-To

Holding on to the pool wall with arms and legs extended (but not locked), pull your knees inward, then return to starting position.

Safety and Alignment Tip

Make a conscious effort to draw in your abdomen during this exercise, but take care not to hold your breath as you do so.

Stretch

Afterward, perform Reaching for the Sky (move #117).

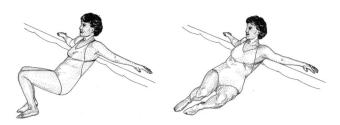

Move #105: The Pool Wall Leg Turn

How-To

1. Holding on to the pool wall with your arms extended (but not locked) and knees bent, alternately turn your legs toward one side and then toward the other side.
2. Keep your knees close to your chest as you move.

Safety and Alignment Tip

Make a conscious effort to draw in your abdomen during this exercise, but take care not to hold your breath as you do so.

Stretch

Afterward, perform the Hip Turn (move #122).

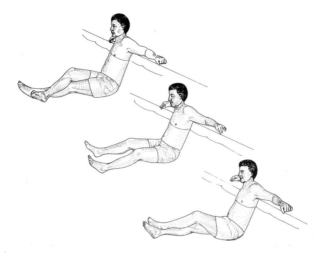

Move #106: The Leg Scissor

How-To

Holding on to the pool wall with your arms and legs extended (but not locked), alternately scissor one leg across the other.

Safety and Alignment Tip

Make a conscious effort to draw in your abdomen during this exercise, but take care not to hold your breath as you do so.

Stretch

Afterward, perform the Sea Stretch (move #123).

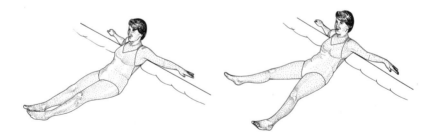

Move #107: Legs Together and Apart

How-To

Holding on to the pool wall with your arms and legs extended (but not locked), alternate spreading your legs apart and then drawing them together.

Safety and Alignment Tip

Make a conscious effort to draw in your abdomen during this exercise, but take care not to hold your breath as you do so.

Stretch

Afterward, perform the Sea Stretch (move #123).

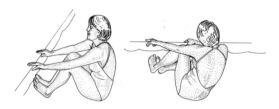

Move #108: Swinging the Buttocks

How-To

Holding on to the pool wall with your elbows and knees bent, place both feet on the wall directly below your hands. Alternately swing your hips to one side above the water's surface and then to the other side.

Stretch

Afterward, perform the Sea Stretch (move #123).

Lower Body

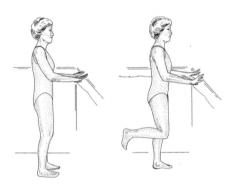

Move #109: The Buttocks and Hamstring Firmer

How-To

Use the pool wall as a ballet barre: Touch the wall for balance, but do not lean on it. Perform leg lifts, bending your knee and raising your foot toward the back.

Safety and Alignment Tips

1. Remember to keep your back straight, and relax your elbows as well as the knee of the leg that is supporting your weight.
2. Be careful not to overbend during lifts, creating a pulling sensation in or around the knee.

Stretch

Afterward, perform the Wet Leg-Hug Stretch (move #124).

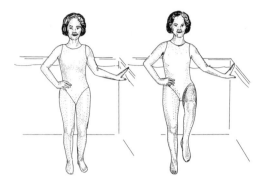

Move #110: The Quadriceps Firmer

How-To

Use the pool wall as a ballet barre: Touch the wall for balance, but do not lean on it. Perform bent-knee leg lifts to the front.

Safety and Alignment Tip

Remember to keep your back straight, and relax your elbow as well as the knee of the leg that is supporting your weight.

Stretch

Afterward, perform the Lift to the Back Stretch (move #125).

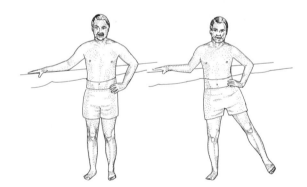

Move #111: The Outer Thigh Firmer

How-To

Use the pool wall as a ballet barre: Touch the wall for balance, but do not lean on it. Perform leg lifts to the side.

Safety and Alignment Tips

1. Don't try to lift too high. Be sure to relax the knee of your working leg. Try to keep the outside of your leg and the outside of your foot facing outward and upward.
2. Remember to keep your back straight, and relax your elbow as well as the knee of the leg that is supporting your weight.

Variation

For an easier, more stress-free version (or simply for variety's sake), perform bent-knee lifts.

Stretch

Afterward, perform the Stretch-Over (move #126).

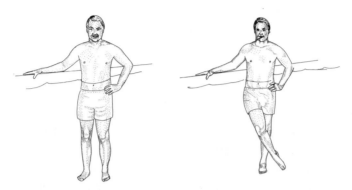

Move #112: The Inner Thigh Firmer

How-To

Use the pool wall as a ballet barre: Touch the wall for balance, but do not lean on it. Perform leg lifts inward (toward the central axis of your body) in front of the other leg.

Safety and Alignment Tips

1. Don't try to lift too high. If the working hip is *arthritic*, do not lift past the midline of your body. Be sure to relax the knee of your working leg. Try to keep the inside of your leg and the inside of your foot facing inward and upward.
2. Remember to keep your back straight, and relax your elbow as well as the knee of the leg that is supporting your weight.

Stretch

Afterward, perform the Shift Stretch (move #127).

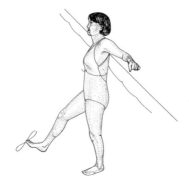

Move #113: The Figure Eight With Foot

How-To

Without moving your leg, draw a figure eight with your toes.

Safety and Alignment Tip

Remember to mind your posture and alignment! Extend both arms to hold the pool wall, but do not lean against it or lock your elbows. Keep your back straight, and relax both knees. Tighten the buttocks and abdomen.

Variation

Draw other numerical and alphabetical figures with your foot.

Stretch

Afterward, perform the Wet Point Stretch (move #128) and the Wet Flex Stretch (move #129).

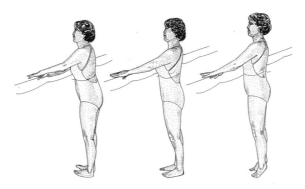

Move #114: Toes Up/Heels Up

How-To

Use the pool wall as a ballet barre: Touch the wall for balance, but do not lean on it. Alternate lifting your toes and then lifting your heels. Between lifts, relax your feet down to the bottom of the pool.

Safety and Alignment Tip
Holding at the front rather than at the back, follow the posture and alignment guidelines suggested for the Figure Eight With Foot (move #113).

Stretch
Afterward, perform the Wet Point Stretch (move #128) and the Wet Flex Stretch (move #129).

Stretches

Upper Body

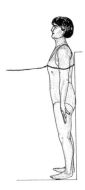

Move #115: The Good Posture Stretch
How-To
1. Stand tall and press your back to the pool wall.
2. Allow your rib cage to elevate. Press your shoulders back and downward by reaching down with your fingers.

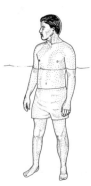

Move #116: The Head Turn
How-To
Perform the Head Turn (move #55) while standing in the pool.
Variation
If you like, you may also perform the Head Tilt (move #56) and the Nod (move #57) in the pool.

Safety and Alignment Tip
Be sure to follow the safety guidelines given with the instructions for these neck movements (moves #55, #56, and #57).

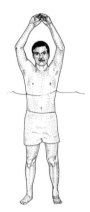

Move #117: Reaching for the Sky

How-To
Remembering to use good posture as described in chapter 3, reach high overhead while loosely holding your hands together.

Variation
If you have trouble reaching high overhead, then simply reach as high as feels natural and comfortable. Or stretch your arms out to the sides at shoulder level.

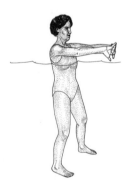

Move #118: The Feel-Good Stretch

How-To
With your fingers intertwined, turn your palms away from your body and stretch your arms toward the front at chest level.

Variation
Your arms may be above, on, or below the water's surface.

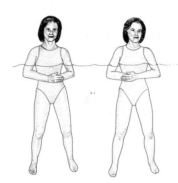

Move #119: Bending at the Wrists

How-To

With your arms submerged, place your hands together, fingertip to fingertip. Begin with your fingers pointing forward. Press gently toward one side. After holding that stretch for a few moments, press gently toward the other side.

Variation

If you like, you may also perform the Steepling Stretch (move #62) and the Turning the Hands Stretch (move #63) in the pool.

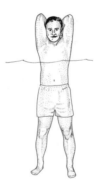

Move #120: The Elbows Up Stretch

How-To

Begin by placing one hand atop the other at the nape of your neck. Slowly slide your hands downward until your elbows point straight up.

Safety and Alignment Tip

Pay special attention to your posture during this exercise. Be careful not to go swayback or lock your knees. Instead, tighten up your buttocks and abdominal muscles, relax the knees, and keep your spine as straight as you can.

Variations
1. If you have trouble pointing your elbows upward, then simply perform your best version of this stretch.
2. If you like, you may also perform the Stretch-Across (move #58) or the Big Stretch (move #59) in the pool.

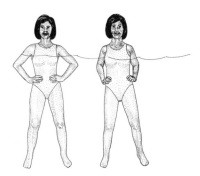

Move #121: The Elbows Backward Stretch

How-To

With your hands on your hips, gently direct your elbows rearward.

Safety and Alignment Tip

Mind your posture as in the Elbows Up Stretch (move #120).

Variation

If you like, you may also perform the Chest Stretcher (move #64), the Bent Stretch (move #65) or the Shoulder-Touch Stretch (move #66) in the pool.

Midsection

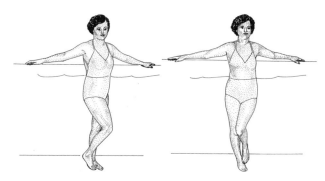

Move #122: The Hip Turn

How-To
1. Standing with your back to the pool wall, hold on to the wall with your arms extended (but not locked). Gently turn your

hips as far as possible toward one side. After holding that stretch for a few moments, gently turn your hips toward the other side.

2. Keep your upper body facing forward throughout these stretches.

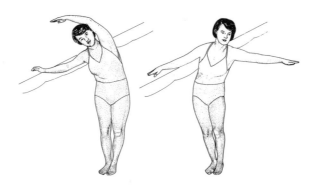

Move #123: The Sea Stretch
How-To
1. Stand with your side to the wall and your feet together at arm's length from the wall. Hold the wall with your arm extended (but not locked). As you pull your hips away from the wall, reach inward with the outside arm over your head. After holding that stretch for a few moments, pull your hips toward the wall and stretch the arm downward and outward.
2. After performing these stretches, be sure to turn and face the opposite direction. Repeat with your second side to the wall.

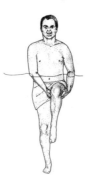

Move #124: The Wet Leg-Hug Stretch
How-To
Give yourself a hug—you deserve it!

Safety and Alignment Tip

Be sure to place your hands on your thigh behind the knee, not around the knee. And remember to relax the knee of the leg that is supporting your weight.

Variation

You may stand with your back on the pool wall for balance. Or when you grow sufficiently confident, try this stretch without touching the wall, to promote your sense of balance.

Lower Body

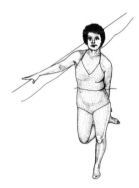

Move #125: The Lift to the Back Stretch

How-To

With your side to the pool wall, touch the wall for balance. Bend the inside leg rearward and upward at the knee.

Safety and Alignment Tips

1. You need not perform a severe knee bend to elongate the quadriceps. If you feel a pulling sensation in or around your knee, you are bending too far. Decrease the degree of your bend.

2. You may hold the lifted heel with your outside hand. It is easier to reach the heel than it is to reach the top of the foot. In fact, it is not necessary to hold at all, and forcing yourself to do so could result in overbending the knee. Employ that technique only if you can do so with relative ease, without experiencing a pulling sensation in or around your knee, and if you feel that it helps your leg to relax into the stretch. If you have trouble reaching your heel, then simply lift your foot to the back without holding.

3. Remember to relax the knee of the leg that is supporting your weight.

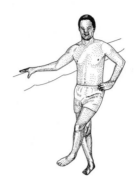

Move #126: The Stretch-Over
How-To
With your side to the pool wall, touch the wall for balance. Cross your outside leg over the inside leg far enough to feel a pleasant stretch in the outer thigh region.
Safety and Alignment Tip
Remember to relax the knee of the leg that is supporting your weight.

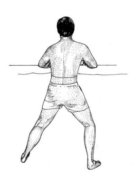

Move #127: The Shift Stretch
How-To
Face the wall, holding on with both hands. Begin by placing your feet as far apart as is comfortable. Shift your hips toward the side, causing one leg to bend and the other to stretch.
Safety and Alignment Tip
Remember to keep your elbows relaxed.

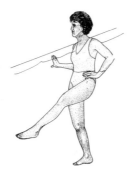

Move #128: The Wet Point Stretch

How-To
Touching the pool wall for balance, extend your leg and point the toe.

Safety and Alignment Tip
Remember to relax your elbow as well as the knee of the leg that is supporting your weight.

Variation
When you grow sufficiently confident, you may try this stretch without touching the wall, to promote your sense of balance.

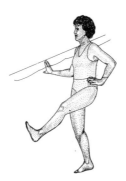

Move #129: The Wet Flex Stretch

How-To
Touching the pool wall for balance, extend your leg and flex the foot.

Safety and Alignment Tip
The tip given along with the Wet Point Stretch (move #128) also applies to this stretch.

Variation
The variation suggested with the Wet Point Stretch (move #128) also applies to this stretch.

PART III

PUTTING IT ALL TOGETHER

CHAPTER 8

Plans and Options

As you have seen from the previous chapters, many approaches can be taken to achieve effective fitness programming. The mature exerciser may enjoy almost any combination of active leisure pastimes, aerobic exercise, muscle conditioning work, and stretch—all to his or her healthful benefit. And all forms of exercise may be accomplished either on land or in the pool!

Near the beginning of this book you were encouraged to please yourself by designing a Full Life exercise plan suitable to your personal tastes, physical needs, and time commitment opportunities. In structuring such a plan, keep in mind that aerobic exercise should be performed at least three times a week, spaced out over the course of each week, whenever possible. For the greatest improvements, calisthenic exercise also should be performed three times per week, if possible. Stretch should accompany other forms of exercise and also can be performed separately.

Mature adults should limit vigorous exercise to not more than 5 days per week—although most adults can safely pursue active leisure pastimes daily, and many can enjoy active hobbies without undue fatigue even on days when structured exercise is also performed. The length of energetic exercise sessions should not exceed 1 hour apiece. With those guidelines in mind, you can use the information in this book to develop a truly personalized Full Life program.

Calendars 8.1 through 8.12 provide samples of practical 3-day, 4-day, and 5-day workout plans designed to promote general fitness.

Let's break down our options even more specifically. For example, a general 5-day land-only plan might be devised as in Calendar 8.13.

Alternatively, a 5-day program for basic fitness with a focus on increased flexibility might work like the program in Calender 8.14.

Calendar 8.15 presents yet another option, a basic land-and-water 5-day plan.

To demonstrate the variety of combinations available, Calendar 8.16 lists an entire month's worth of sample Full Life activities on a basic 5-day plan.

If you grow quite fit—and chances are good that you will—you may eventually opt to include both aerobic and calisthenic work 4 to 5 days per week. But you should certainly build up to that very gradually.

Remember that when similar workouts are undertaken during the same week, you can still enjoy variety. For example, if you perform low-impact aerobic dance on land every Monday, Wednesday, and Friday, you can vary your movement sequences and combinations from session to session. You also can change musical selections as often as you like.

The same principle holds true with stretch and calisthenic work as well as with all forms of exercise performed in water. As demonstrated in the sample fitness plans, you also may vary active leisure pursuits. Change your routine as often as you like! If you are one of those people who thrives on regularity, frequent changes may be unnecessary. You may enjoy the sense of security that comes with following an established program. For example, a daily stroll with your cocker spaniel may completely satisfy your active leisure needs. But if variety is important to you—and it may grow increasingly so as your fitness level advances—then partake of a diverse assortment of fitness activities and training methods. Don't forget that you can introduce both aerobic and strength-training exercise machines into your Full Life Fitness plan, if you desire.

CALENDAR 8.1

Three-Day Plan No. 1

Sunday:	Monday:	Tuesday:	Wednesday:	Thursday:	Friday:	Saturday:
Rest (or active leisure pastime)	Total-body pool workout	Rest (or active leisure pastime)	Total-body pool workout	Rest (or active leisure pastime)	Total-body pool workout	Rest (or active leisure pastime)

CALENDAR 8.2

Three-Day Plan No. 2

Sunday:	Monday:	Tuesday:	Wednesday:	Thursday:	Friday:	Saturday:
Rest (or active leisure pastime)	Total-body land workout	Rest (or active leisure pastime)	Total-body land workout	Rest (or active leisure pastime)	Total-body land workout	Rest (or active leisure pastime)

CALENDAR 8.3

Three-Day Plan No. 3

Sunday:	Monday:	Tuesday:	Wednesday:	Thursday:	Friday:	Saturday:
Rest (or active leisure pastime)	Total-body pool workout	Rest (or active leisure pastime)	Total-body land workout	Rest (or active leisure pastime)	Total-body pool workout	Rest (or active leisure pastime)

CALENDAR 8.4

Three-Day Plan No. 4

Sunday:	Monday:	Tuesday:	Wednesday:	Thursday:	Friday:	Saturday:
Rest (or active leisure pastime)	Total-body land workout	Rest (or active leisure pastime)	Total-body pool workout	Rest (or active leisure pastime)	Total-body land workout	Rest (or active leisure pastime)

CALENDAR 8.5

Four-Day Plan No. 1

Sunday:	Monday:	Tuesday:	Wednesday:	Thursday:	Friday:	Saturday:
Rest (or active leisure pastime)	Total-body pool workout	Rest (or active leisure pastime)	Total-body pool workout	Rest (or active leisure pastime)	Pool aerobics and stretch	Pool calisthenics and stretch

CALENDAR 8.6

Four-Day Plan No. 2

Sunday:	Monday:	Tuesday:	Wednesday:	Thursday:	Friday:	Saturday:
Rest (or active leisure pastime)	Total-body land workout	Rest (or active leisure pastime)	Total-body land workout	Rest (or active leisure pastime)	Land aerobics and stretch	Land calisthenics and stretch

CALENDAR 8.7

Four-Day Plan No. 3

Sunday:	Monday:	Tuesday:	Wednesday:	Thursday:	Friday:	Saturday:
Rest (or active leisure pastime)	Total-body pool workout	Rest (or active leisure pastime)	Total-body land workout	Rest (or active leisure pastime)	Pool aerobics and stretch	Land calisthenics and stretch

CALENDAR 8.8

Four-Day Plan No. 4

Sunday:	Monday:	Tuesday:	Wednesday:	Thursday:	Friday:	Saturday:
Rest (or active leisure pastime)	Total-body pool workout	Rest (or active leisure pastime)	Total-body land workout	Rest (or active leisure pastime)	Land aerobics and stretch	Pool calisthenics and stretch

CALENDAR 8.9

Five-Day Plan No. 1

Sunday:	Monday:	Tuesday:	Wednesday:	Thursday:	Friday:	Saturday:
Rest (or active leisure pastime)	Pool aerobics and stretch	Pool calisthenics and stretch	Pool aerobics, calisthenics, and stretch	Rest (or active leisure pastime)	Pool aerobics and stretch	Pool calisthenics and stretch

CALENDAR 8.10

Five-Day Plan No. 2

Sunday:	Monday:	Tuesday:	Wednesday:	Thursday:	Friday:	Saturday:
Rest (or active leisure pastime)	Land aerobics and stretch	Land calisthenics and stretch	Land aerobics, calisthenics, and stretch	Rest (or active leisure pastime)	Land aerobics and stretch	Land calisthenics and stretch

CALENDAR 8.11

Five-Day Plan No. 3

Sunday:	Monday:	Tuesday:	Wednesday:	Thursday:	Friday:	Saturday:
Rest (or active leisure pastime)	Pool aerobics and stretch	Land calisthenics and stretch	Pool aerobics, calisthenics, and stretch	Rest (or active leisure pastime)	Land aerobics and stretch	Pool calisthenics and stretch

CALENDAR 8.12

Five-Day Plan No. 4

Sunday:	Monday:	Tuesday:	Wednesday:	Thursday:	Friday:	Saturday:
Rest (or active leisure pastime)	Pool aerobics and stretch	Land calisthenics and stretch	Pool aerobics, calisthenics, and stretch	Rest (or active leisure pastime)	Pool aerobics and stretch	Land calisthenics and stretch

CALENDAR 8.13

Five-Day Plan No. 5: A Varied Land-Only Program

Sunday:	Monday:	Tuesday:	Wednesday:	Thursday:	Friday:	Saturday:
Rest (or active leisure pastime)	Stationary cycling and stretch	Calisthenics and stretch	Brisk walking, calisthenics, and stretch	Rest (or active leisure pastime)	Low-impact aerobic dance and stretch	Calisthenics and stretch

CALENDAR 8.14

Five-Day Plan No. 6: A Stretch-Oriented Program

Sunday:	Monday:	Tuesday:	Wednesday:	Thursday:	Friday:	Saturday:
Rest (or active leisure pastime)	Pool aerobics, calisthenics, and stretch	Stretch-only on land	Rest (or active leisure pastime)	Low-impact aerobic dance on land, calisthenics, and stretch	Stretch-only in pool	Stationary cycling and stretch

CALENDAR 8.15

Five-Day Plan No. 7: A Varied Land and Pool Program

Sunday:	Monday:	Tuesday:	Wednesday:	Thursday:	Friday:	Saturday:
Rest (or active leisure pastime)	Pool aerobics and stretch	Land calisthenics and stretch	Brisk walking on land, calisthenics, and stretch	Rest (or active leisure pastime)	Bicycling around town and stretch	Pool calisthenics and stretch

CALENDAR 8.16

A Month in the Full Life

Sunday	Monday	Tuesday	Wednesday	Thursday	Friday	Saturday
1st Day: Rest	2nd Day: Pool aerobics and stretch	3rd Day: Land calisthenics and stretch	4th Day: Gardening as an active leisure activity	5th Day: Pool aerobics, calisthenics, and stretch	6th Day: Pool calisthenics and stretch	7th Day: Stationary cycling and stretch
8th Day: Rest	9th Day: Brisk walking on land and stretch	10th Day: Pool calisthenics and stretch	11th Day: Ballroom dance as an active leisure activity	12th Day: Pool aerobics, calisthenics, and stretch	13th Day (!): Land calisthenics and stretch	14th Day: Low-impact aerobic dance on land and stretch
15th Day: Rest	16th Day: Pool aerobics and stretch	17th Day: Land calisthenics and stretch	18th Day: Walking nine holes of golf as an active leisure activity	19th Day: Brisk walking on land, calisthenics, and stretch	20th Day: Pool calisthenics and stretch	21st Day: Pool aerobics and stretch
22nd Day: Rest	23rd Day: Bicycle around town and stretch	24th Day: Pool calisthenics and stretch	25th Day: Shopping or sightseeing as an active leisure activity	26th Day: Pool aerobics, calisthenics, and stretch	27th Day: Land calisthenics and stretch	28th Day: Pool aerobics and stretch
29th Day: Rest	30th Day: Pool aerobics and stretch	31st Day: Land calisthenics and stretch				

In leading your Full Life, remember the following rules for success:

1. Very light exercise is almost always better than *no* exercise. If you have been sedentary, you will even benefit from simply adopting an active leisure pastime (as described in chapter 1) and pursuing it faithfully.
2. When you are getting started, it is perfectly acceptable to perform low-intensity or short-duration exercise to build up your endurance and strength. So do not worry about reaching your training heart rate or performing aerobic exercise for 20 to 30 minutes continuously until you are fit enough to meet those criteria without overdoing things. Progress slowly.
3. Reduce the challenge of your workout if it results in over-fatigue. Follow chapter 3's guidelines for "backing off" and for gradually building back up again.
4. Likewise, follow the instructions given throughout this book for preventing undue soreness, unnecessary exercise-related injuries, and overexertion.
5. Use the sample plans given in this chapter, or institute a personalized plan of your own based on the guidelines of the Full Life exercise program.
6. Enjoy as narrow or as broad a range of activities as appeals to you.
7. Seek pleasure through movement. Instead of simply tackling drills, undertake physical activities that provide satisfaction. Pursue them to an extent at which they improve personal health and increase your enjoyment of living.

CHAPTER 9

Sticking With It for the Best of Your Life

To achieve the Full Life, you must make physical exercise a stable aspect of your weekly routine. Exercise cannot yield the lasting physiological benefits you deserve if it is only performed every now and then—for instance, when you want to lose a few pounds—and then abandoned. It cannot provide enduring mental and emotional rewards if it is undertaken sporadically. In other words, exercise should not be viewed as a "quick fix" to be applied only on especially stressful days.

It takes regular exercise performed on a continuing basis to (a) promote the flexibility and strength needed for preserving optimal mobility in later years, (b) produce major psychological benefits such as higher morale and improved self-image, and (c) keep a body fit and energized for enjoying life to its fullest!

But chances are that by this point you do not need much convincing that regular exercise is desirable. You may well be more concerned about the challenge of *sticking with your exercise program* once it is under way. Perhaps you have fallen away from fitness regimes in the past and you could use some practical advice for keeping yourself motivated. Table 9.1 gives some suggestions that may help.

TABLE 9.1

Quick Tips for Success
• **Use music.**
• **Create variety.**
• **Seek moderation.**   People who attempt grueling, exhausting workouts tend to drop out sooner than those who adopt lighter regimens.
• **Seek convenience.**   Think twice before joining a health club that is located more than a few minutes' drive from your home or workplace. Owning a variety of workout videos can be a very handy convenience for club members and outdoor exercisers when the car is under repair, for example, or when it is raining.
• **Set up a schedule.**   It is better to set aside a certain time of day for exercise than it is to try to fit workouts in around other activities without a planned schedule.
• **Exercise with a partner.**   Partners provide an atmosphere of mutual support and inspire long-term adherence. When an individual partner is not available, joining a group exercise program offers similar benefits. Social opportunities can make exercise more fun, and exercise activities can, in turn, create social opportunities! So consider exercise avenues that may trigger just that type of positive "vicious circle."

USING SELF-PSYCHOLOGY

In his book *The Exercise Habit,* sport psychologist James Gavin explores the psychoemotional dynamics involved in determining whether an individual will be successful in making exercise a permanent and regular part of life. Gavin's approach to exercise adherence stresses the importance of maintaining a high state of awareness as to *why* one has chosen to pursue an active lifestyle in the first place. Toward this end, it is useful to set reasonable short-range goals (for example, realistic weight-loss goals). Mastering the proper methods for achieving these goals can, of course, help prevent discouragement after one's exercise program is undertaken. But more importantly, one must also acknowledge those most basic personal desires that underlie the cognitive intention to exercise.

The Full Life Fitness program equips you to approach short-range goals in a practical and effective manner. The previous chapters of this book have explained which types of exercise regimens are best for losing body fat, for improving flexibility, for building strength, and for tackling other projects such as increasing energy levels and managing day-to-day stress.

In establishing personal short-range goals, do try not to be too hard on yourself. Remember that it will take time to get into shape—just as it has taken time to get *out* of shape! Allow yourself the weeks or months necessary for physical training effects to become evident. And in the meantime, don't fail to give yourself a pat on the back after each scheduled exercise session you complete. Remind yourself that every workout accomplished represents one more step you have taken in the right direction!

The desire to lead a truly full and rewarding life is one example of the type of fundamental urge that might move a person to begin exercising regularly and then sustain that person in maintaining a consistent exercise program for life. Another example might be the hope of living a long and healthy life. And still another might be the need to feel in possession of personal self-control. We are talking about the strongest personal passion that maintaining an exercise lifestyle can help one to satisfy.

Naturally, this powerful source of strength and discipline will vary from person to person. So take some time to consider the long-term dreams that regular exercise can help to fulfill in *your* life. Condense your thoughts into a "nutshell"—into one short statement that sums up why you should make exercise a lifelong habit. Bring this thought to mind on days when you do not feel motivated to work out. It may just be the key that gets you going and *keeps* you going for life.

Remember that with Full Life Fitness you never should force yourself to continue an activity you detest or find unpleasantly boring—or even one you have simply grown tired of! Indeed, a major premise of the Full Life program is that if you are not enjoying something about your fitness activities, then those particular activities are not right for you. So be adventurous! If one physical undertaking disappoints you, then shelve it and try another. With so many forms of exercise, so many types of sport and dance, and so many active leisure pastimes available to you, there is no reason to settle for something that is less than satisfying. And needless to say, the more pleasure any pursuit affords you, the greater your likelihood is of keeping at it.

Along these same lines, you may ultimately find it constructive to "baby" yourself every once in a while. For example, let us say that Wednesday is one of your aerobics days and you haven't missed a scheduled session for months. But for some inexplicable reason, when this Wednesday rolls around, you just cannot seem to get yourself started. Even after you have reminded yourself of the purpose of exercise in your life, something in your mental makeup resists the idea of performing your workout. In this special situation, you have actually earned the right to consider giving yourself a bit of a break. Do not skip your exercise period altogether. But do permit yourself the flexibility of substituting an alternate activity that strikes you at the time as more appealing. You might, for example, simply enjoy a nice walk outdoors, perform a stretch-only routine on land or in the pool, or busy yourself with an active leisure pastime that is sure to please.

In getting down to basics about the psychological incentives you can draw on to succeed at an exercise lifestyle, wellness writer Sherman Dickson made a good point by noting that to sustain activity over time, one must discover and undertake activity that is stimulating and enjoyable.

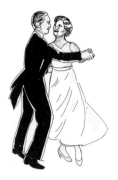

LOOKING AT YOUR OVERALL LIFESTYLE

Remember that exercise alone cannot ensure optimal health. Adopting good-sense lifestyle habits, such as following a well-balanced diet, increases one's potential for success in any fitness program. Feeling successful increases the pleasure one derives from exercise activity and increases one's enthusiasm for further physical movement. Conquering *negative* lifestyle habits, like cigarette smoking, contributes toward the same desirable outcomes. Attending to overall health care matters in cooperation with a qualified personal physician completes the picture. Combine these practical measures with an enjoyable Full Life exercise plan, and you will be well on your way toward the achievement of lasting good looks and good health.

You have the power to succeed at physical fitness and to continue enjoying the benefits of regular exercise for a lifetime. So, be *good* to yourself. Commit once and for all to living the Full Life!

Bibliography

Albanes, D., Blair, A., & Taylor, P.R. (1989). Physical activity and risk of cancer in the NHANES I population. *American Journal of Public Health*, **79**(6), 744-750.

American Heart Association. (1983). *An older person's guide to cardiovascular health*. Dallas: Author.

Aniansson, A., & Gustafsson, E. (1981). Physical training in elderly men with special reference to quadriceps muscle strength and morphology. *Clinical Physiology*, **1**, 87-98.

Avers, D., & Wharton, M.A. (1991). Improving exercise adherence: Instructional strategies. *Topics in Geriatric Rehabilitation*, **6**(3), 62-73.

Barndt, R., Blankenhorn, D., Crawford, D., & Brooks, S. (1977). Regression and progression of early femoral atherosclerosis in treated hyperlipoproteinemic patients. *Annals of Internal Medicine*, **86**(2), 139-146.

Bell, R.D., & Laskin, J. (1985). The use of curl-up variations in the development of abdominal musculature strength and endurance by post 50-year-old volunteers. *Journal of Human Movement Studies*, **11**(6), 319-324.

Beverly, M.C., Rider, T.A., Evans, M.J., & Smith, R. (1989). Local bone mineral response to brief exercise that stresses the skeleton. *British Medical Journal*, **299**(6693), 233-237.

Biegel, L. (1984). *Physical fitness and the older person: A guide to exercise for health care professionals*. Rockville, MD: Aspen Systems Corporation.

Blair, S.N., Kohl, H.W., III, Paffenbarger, R.S., Jr., Clark, D.G., Cooper, K.H., & Gibbons, L.W. (1989). Physical fitness and all-cause mortality: A prospective study of healthy men and women. *Journal of the American Medical Association*, **262**(17), 2395-2401.

Blumenthal, J.A., Emery, C.F., Madden, D.J., George, L.K., Coleman, R.E., Riddle, M.W., McKee, D.C., Reasoner, J., & Williams, R.S. (1989). Cardiovascular and behavioral effects of aerobic exercise training in healthy older men and women. *Journal of Gerontology*, **44**(5), 147-157.

Blumenthal, J.A., Fredrikson, M., Kuhn, C.M., Ulmer, R.L., Walsh-Riddle, M., & Appelbaum, M. (1990). Aerobic exercise reduces levels of cardiovascular and sympathoadrenal responses to mental stress in subjects without prior evidence of myocardial ischemia. *American Journal of Cardiology*, **65**(1), 93-98.

Borg, G.A.V. (1982). Psychophysical bases of perceived exertion. *Medicine and Science in Sports and Exercise*, **14**, 377-381.

Boyer, J., & Kasch, F. (1970). Exercise therapy in hypertensive men. *Journal of the American Medical Association*, **211**, 1668-1671.

Burke, W.E., Tuttle, W.W., Thompson, C.W., Janney, C.D., & Weber, R.J. (1953). The relation of grip strength and grip-strength endurance to age. *Journal of Applied Physiology*, **5**, 628-630.

Campbell, M.J., McComas, A.J., & Petito, F. (1973). Physiological changes in ageing muscles. *Journal of Neurology, Neurosurgery, and Psychiatry*, **36**, 174-182.

Carter, D.R. (1984). Mechanical loading histories and cortical bone remodeling. *Calcified Tissue International*, **36**, S19-S24.

Chapman, E.A., deVries, H.A., & Sweezey, R. (1972). Joint stiffness and effects of exercise on young and old men. *Journal of Gerontology*, **27**(2), 218-221.

Coats, A.J., Adamopoulos, S., Meyer, T.E., Conway, J., & Sleight, P. (1990). Effects of physical training in chronic heart failure. *Lancet*, **335**(8681), 63-66.

Collins, K.J., & Exton-Smith, A.N. (1983). Thermal homeostasis in old age. *Journal of the American Geriatrics Society*, **31**, 519-524.

Dannenberg, A.L., Keller, J.B., Wilson, P.W., & Castelli, W.P. (1989). Leisure time physical activity in the Framingham Offspring Study: Description, seasonal variation, and risk factor correlates. *American Journal of Epidemiology*, **129**(1), 76-88.

deVries, H.A., & Adams, G.M. (1972). Electromyographic comparison of single doses of exercises and meprobamate as to effects on muscular relaxation. *American Journal of Physical Medicine, 51,* 140-148.

Dickson, S.R. (1988). *Pathways to wellness.* Champaign, IL: Human Kinetics.

Ekelund, L.G., Haskell, W.L., Johnson, J.L., Whaley, F.S., Criqui, M.H., & Sheps, D.S. (1988). Physical fitness as a predictor of cardiovascular mortality in asymptomatic North American men: The Lipid Research Clinics mortality follow-up study. *New England Journal of Medicine, 319*(21), 1379-1384.

Ewart, C.K., Stewart, K.J., Gillilan, R.E., & Kelemen, M.H. (1986). Self-efficacy mediates strength gains during circuit weight training in men with coronary artery disease. *Medicine and Science in Sports and Exercise, 18*(2), 531-540.

Fiataroni, M.A., Marks, E.C., Ryan, N.D., Meredith, C.N., Lipsitz, L.A., & Evans, W.J. (1990). High-intensity strength training in nonagenarians: Effects on skeletal muscle. *Journal of the American Medical Association, 263*(22), 3029-3034.

Gavin, J. (1992). *The exercise habit.* Champaign, IL: Human Kinetics.

Glickstein, J.K., & White, J.F. (Eds.) (1990). Putting the problem in perspective. *Focus on Geriatric Care & Rehabilitation, 3*(9), 1.

Greer, M., Dimick, S., & Burns, S. (1984). Heart rate and blood pressure response to several methods of strength training. *Physical Therapy, 64*(1), 179-183.

Greist, J.H., Klein, M.H., Eischens, R.R., & Faris, J.T. (1978). Running out of depression. *Physician and Sportsmedicine, 6,* 49-56.

Gulton, L. (1975). *Don't give up on an aging patient.* New York: Crown.

Hamilton, E.N.M., & Whitney, E.N. (1982). *Nutrition: Concepts and controversies (2nd ed.).* St. Paul, MN: West.

Hardman, A.E., Hudson, A., Jones, P.R.M., & Norgan, N.G. (1989). Brisk walking and plasma high density lipoprotein cholesterol concentration in previously sedentary women. *British Medical Journal, 299*(6709), 1204-1205.

Harris, L. (1978). *Aging in the eighties: America in transition.* Washington, DC: National Council on the Aging.

Hubert, H.B., Feinleib, M., McNamara, R.M., & Castelli, W.P. (1983). Obesity as an independent risk factor for cardiovascular disease: A 26-year follow-up of participants in the Framingham heart study. *Circulation, 67,* 968-977.

Johns Hopkins Medical Institutions. (1990a). Making the heart stronger. *The Johns Hopkins Medical Letter: Health After 50, 1*(12), 1.

Johns Hopkins Medical Institutions. (1990b). Should you have an exercise stress test? *The Johns Hopkins Medical Letter: Health After 50*, **2**(8), 7.

Kauffman, T. (1990). Impact of aging-related musculoskeletal and postural changes on falls. *Topics in Geriatric Rehabilitation*, **5**(2), 34-43.

Kelemen, M.H., Effron, M.B., Valenti, S.A., & Stewart, K.J. (1990). Exercise training combined with antihypertensive drug therapy: Effects on lipids, blood pressure, and left ventricular mass. *Journal of the American Medical Association*, **263**(20), 2766-2771.

Kelemen, M.H., Stewart, K.J., Gillilan, R.E., Ewart, C.K., Valenti, S.A., Manley, J.D., & Kelemen, M.D. (1986). Circuit weight training in cardiac patients. *Journal of the American College of Cardiology*, **7**(1), 38-42.

Kelly, S.S. (1978). The effect of age on neuromuscular transmission. *Journal of Physiology*, **274**, 51-62.

Kreindler, H., Lewis, C.B., Rush, S., & Schaefer, K. (1989). Effects of three exercise protocols on strength of persons with osteoarthritis of the knee. *Topics in Geriatric Rehabilitation*, **4**(3), 32-39.

Kuta, I., Parizkova, J., & Dycka, J. (1970). Muscle strength and lean body mass in old men of different physical activity. *Journal of Applied Physiology*, **29**(2), 168-171.

LaForest, S., St-Perre, D.M.M., Cyr, J., & Gayton, D. (1990). Effects of age and regular exercise on muscle strength and endurance. *European Journal of Applied Physiology*, **60**, 104-111.

Larsson, L. (1982). Physical training effects on muscle morphology in sedentary males at different ages. *Medicine and Science in Sports and Exercise*, **14**(3), 203-206.

Larsson, L., Grimby, G., & Karlsson, J. (1979). Muscle strength and speed of movement in relation to age and muscle morphology. *Journal of Applied Physiology*, **46**(3), 451-456.

Leslie, D.R., & Frekany, G.A. (1975). Effects of an exercise program on selected flexibility measures of senior citizens. *Gerontologist*, **4**, 182-183.

Lutwak, L. (1969). Symposium on osteoporosis: Nutritional aspects of osteoporosis. *Journal of the American Geriatrics Society*, **17**(2), 115-119.

Michel, B.A., Block, D.A., & Fries, J.F. (1989). Weight-bearing exercise, overexercise, and lumbar bone density over age 50 years. *Archives of Internal Medicine*, **149**(7), 2325-2329.

Milesis, C.A., Pollock, M.L., Bah, M.D., Ayres, J.J., Ward, A., & Linnerud, A.C. (1976). Effects of different durations of training on cardiorespiratory function, body composition and serum liquids. *Research Quarterly, 47,* 716-725.

Morey, M.C., Cowper, P.A., Feussner, J.R., DiPasquale, R.C., Crowley, G.M., Kitzman, D.W., & Sullivan, R.J., Jr. (1989). Evaluation of a supervised exercise program in a geriatric population. *Journal of the American Geriatrics Society, 37*(4), 348-354.

Moritani, T., & deVries, H. (1980). Potential for gross muscle hypertrophy in older men. *Journal of Gerontology, 35,* 672-682.

Nakamura, E., Moritani, T., & Kanetaka, A. (1989). Biological age versus physical fitness age. *European Journal of Applied Physiology, 58*(7), 778-785.

Orlander, J., & Aniansson, A. (1980). Effects of physical training on skeletal muscle metabolism and ultrastructure in 70 to 75 year old men. *Acta Physiological Scandinavica, 109,* 149-154.

Paffenbarger, R.S., Hyde, R.T., Wing, A.L., & Hsieh, C. (1986). Physical activity, all-cause mortality, and longevity of college alumni. *New England Journal of Medicine, 314*(10), 605-613.

Pandolf, K.B. (1982). Differentiated ratings of perceived exertion during physical exercise. *Medicine and Science in Sports and Exercise, 14,* 397-405.

Pollock, M.L., Broida, J., Kendrick, Z., Miller, H.S., Janeway, R., & Linnerud, A.C. (1972). Effects of training two days per week at different intensities on middle-aged men. *Medicine and Science in Sports, 4,* 192-197.

Pollock, M.L., Cureton, T.K., & Greninger, L. (1969). Effects of frequency of training on working capacity, cardiovascular function, and body composition of adult men. *Medicine and Science in Sports, 1,* 70-74.

Pollock, M.L., Dawson, G.A., Miller, H.S., Jr., Ward, A., Cooper, D., Headley, W., Linnerud, A.C., & Nomeir, M.M. (1976). Physiologic responses of men 49 to 65 years of age to endurance training. *Journal of the American Geriatrics Society, 24,* 97-104.

Pollock, M.L., Dimmick, J., Miller, H.S., Kendrick, Z., & Linnerud, A.C. (1975). Effects of mode of training on cardiovascular function and body composition of middle-aged men. *Medicine and Science in Sports, 7,* 139-145.

Pollock, M.L., Gettman, L.R., Milesis, C.A., Bah, M.D., Durstine, J.L., & Johnson, R.B. (1977). Effects of frequency and duration of training on attrition and incidence of injury. *Medicine and Science in Sports*, **9**, 31-36.

Reddan, W. (1985). Body fluid and thermal regulation with age. *Topics in Geriatric Rehabilitation*, **1**(1), 40-48.

Serfass, R.C., Agre, J.C., & Smith, E.L. (1985). Exercise testing for the elderly. *Topics in Geriatric Rehabilitation*, **1**(1), 58-67.

Sharkey, B.J. (1970). Intensity and duration of training and the development of cardiorespiratory endurance. *Medicine and Science in Sports*, **2**, 197-202.

Sharkey, B.J., & Holleman, J.P. (1967). Cardiorespiratory adaptations to training at specified intensities. *Research Quarterly*, **38**, 698-704.

Sidney, K.H., Shephard, R.J., & Harrison, J.E. (1977). Endurance training and body composition of the elderly. *American Journal of Clinical Nutrition*, **30**, 326-333.

Skinner, J.S., Hutsler, R., Bergsteinova, V., & Buskirk, E.R. (1973a). Perception of effort during different types of exercise and under different environmental conditions. *Medicine and Science in Sports*, **5**, 110-115.

Skinner, J.S., Hutsler, R., Bergsteinova, V., & Buskirk, E.R. (1973b). The validity and reliability of a rating scale of perceived exertion. *Medicine and Science in Sports*, **5**, 94-96.

Slattery, M.L., Jacobs, D.R., Jr., & Nichaman, M.Z. (1989). Leisure time physical activity and coronary heart disease death: The U.S. railroad study. *Circulation*, **79**(1), 304-311.

Smith, E.L., Reddan, W., & Smith, P.E. (1981). Physical activity and calcium modalities for bone mineral increase in aged women. *Medicine and Science in Sports and Exercise*, **13**(1), 60-64.

Souminen, H.E., Heikkinen, E., & Parkatti, T. (1977). Effect of eight weeks of physical training on muscle and connective tissue on the m. vastus lateralis in 69 year old men and women. *Journal of Gerontology*, **32**, 33-37.

Steinhaus, L.A., Dustman, R.E., Ruhling, R.O., Emmerson, R.Y., Johnson, S.C., Shearer, D.E., Shigeoka, J.W., & Bonekat, W.H. (1988). Cardio-respiratory fitness of young and older active and sedentary men. *British Journal of Sports Medicine*, **22**(4), 163-166.

Tzankoff, S.P., & Norris, A.H. (1977). Effect of muscle mass decrease on age-related BMR changes. *Journal of Applied Physiology*, **43**(6), 1001-1006.

University of Texas Health Science Center at Houston. (1990a). Exercise boosts body's clot busters. *Lifetime Health Letter*, **2**(3), 8.

University of Texas Health Science Center at Houston. (1990b). Short bouts of exercise improve fitness. *Lifetime Health Letter*, 2(6), 8.

U.S. Department of Health & Human Services. (1983). *Aqua dynamics: Water exercises are the new way to stay in shape*. Washington, DC: The President's Council on Physical Fitness and Sports.

Wagner, J., & Horvath, S. (1985). Influence of age and gender on human thermoregulatory responses to cold exposures. *Journal of Applied Physiology*, **58**, 180-186.

Wagner, J., Robinson, S., & Marino, R. (1974). Age and temperature regulations in humans in neutral and cold environments. *Journal of Applied Physiology*, 37, 552-565.

Wilmore, J.H., Royce, J., Girandola, R.N., Katch, F.I., & Katch, V.L. (1970). Physiological alterations resulting from a 10-week jogging program. *Medicine and Science in Sports*, **2**, 7-14.

Index

A

Abdominal region, exercises for, 80-83, 93, 102-103
ACE (American Council on Exercise), 23
Achilles tendon, 95, 107-108
Acoustics in safety, 23
ACSM (American College of Sports Medicine), 23
Adams, G.M., 16
Aerobic exercise
  benefits of, 17, 37, 44
  dance movements for, 49-55
  duration of, 40-41, 42, 112, 158
  in exercise plans, 8, 148, 151-157
  frequency for, 40, 41, 42, 112, 147
  intensity of, 28, 38-40, 42, 43, 48, 112, 114-115, 158
  with medical disorders, 43-44, 113
  program for, 45-48
  types of, 38
  warm-up/cool-down for, 25-28, 29, 48, 114, 116
  in water, 43, 112-113, 114, 115, 116, 117, 118-123
  weight control through, 37, 43, 113-114
Aerobics and Fitness Association of America (AFAA), 23
Aging process
  and circulatory system, 11-12
  and exercise, viii, 3
  and flexibility, 91, 94-95
  and musculoskeletal system, 11, 14, 57-58
  and weight control, 15
Albanes, D., 16
Allergies, 28
American College of Sports Medicine (ACSM), 23
American Council on Exercise (ACE), 23
American Heart Association, 15, 37
American Journal of Physical Medicine, 16
Ankle, exercises for, 107-109
Arm, exercises for, 68-75, 100-101
Arthritis
  and aerobic exercise, 43-44, 113
  general exercise benefits for, viii, 15
  and muscle conditioning, 61, 63-64
  and safety, 21
  and stretch exercise, 93
  and water exercise, 113

Asthma
  and safety, 21, 44
  and specific exercise, 44, 64, 92-93, 113
Atherosclerosis, 12
Avers, D., 57

B

Back, exercises for, 61, 76-77, 93, 103-104
Back pain
  general exercise benefits for, viii, 15
  and specific exercise, 44, 62, 93, 113
Ballet, 91-92
Barndt, Robert, 12
Basal metabolic rate, 15
Biceps, exercises for, 63, 71-72, 99
Bicycle, stationary, 25, 27
Biegel, L., 16
Blair, S.N., 5
Blood clots, 14
Blood pressure. *See* Hypertension
Bones, 14-15, 17, 37. *See also* Musculoskeletal system
Breathing, 12-13, 30, 33, 94, 95
British Medical Journal, 13
Buttocks, exercises for, 61, 83-85, 93, 103-104

C

Calf, exercises for, 28, 63, 88-89, 107-108
Calisthenics. *See also* Muscle conditioning
  for abdominals, 80-83
  for arm and shoulder, 67-75
  for back, 76-77
  for chest, 77-79
  in exercise plans, 8, 148, 151-157
  health benefits of, 17
  for lower body, 83-90
  and medical disorders, 61, 64
  programs for, 64-66, 111-112
  safety of, 30
  warm-up/cool-down for, 25-27, 28, 29
  as warm-ups, 26-27
  in water, 115, 117, 125-136
  for weight loss, 43
Cancer, 16, 17
Cardiopulmonary resuscitation (CPR), 23
Cardiovascular disease, 12-13, 17, 20, 43. *See also* Circulatory system
Chest, exercises for, 77-79, 101-102
Cholesterol, 13, 17, 20, 37
Circulatory system, 3, 4-5, 11-14, 17, 25-26. *See also* Aerobic exercise

Clothing in safety, 24
Cool-down. *See* Warm-up/cool-down
Coronary artery disease, 4. *See also*
    Cardiovascular disease; Circulatory
    system
CPR (cardiopulmonary resuscitation), 23
Cross-training, 42-43, 111

D

Dance
    ballet, 91-92
    movements for aerobics, 49-55
    program for aerobics, 45-48
    for warm-ups, 25
Dehydration, 23
Depression, 16, 17
deVries, H.A., 16
Diabetes
    general exercise benefits for, 16, 17
    and safety, 20, 21
    and specific exercise, 44, 64, 113
Dickson, Sherman, 162
Digestion, benefits of exercise for, 16
Dizziness, 30, 32, 45
Don't Give Up on an Aging Patient
    (Gulton), 16
Duration
    of aerobic exercise, 40-41, 42, 112, 158
    of exercise in general, 7, 148, 158
    of muscle conditioning, 59, 60, 66, 112
    and safety, 23, 31
    of stretch exercise, 92, 94, 112
    of warm-up/cool-down, 25, 27, 28, 29
    of water exercise, 112-113

E

Ekelund, C.K., 5
Endurance
    effects of aging on, 11
    general exercise benefits for, 3, 12, 17
    and specific exercise, 43, 57, 59
Energy level, ix, 12, 17, 37, 43, 159
Equipment in safety, 22
Exercise benefits
    through aerobics, 17, 37, 44
    and the aging process, viii, 3
    for circulatory system, 3, 4, 11-14, 17
    for general physical health, vii, 3-6, 16,
        159
    list of, 17
    for mental/emotional health, 16-17, 159
    through muscle conditioning, 57-58, 64,
        65
    for musculoskeletal system, 3, 14-15,
        17, 37, 57-58, 91, 113
    through stretch exercise, 17, 91, 93-94
    through water exercise, 43, 92, 111
    for weight control, vii, ix, 3, 15-16, 17
Exercise environment in safety, 22-24

Exercise Habit, The (Gavin), 161
Exercise instructions
    for aerobic dance movements, 49-55
    for aerobic dance programs, 45-48
    for muscle conditioning of abdominals,
        80-83
    for muscle conditioning of arm and
        shoulder, 67-75
    for muscle conditioning of back, 76-77
    for muscle conditioning of chest, 77-79
    for muscle conditioning of lower body,
        83-90
    for muscle conditioning programs,
        64-66
    for resistance training programs, 59-60,
        61, 62
    for stretch exercise programs, 94-95
    for stretching back and lower body,
        103-109
    for stretching upper body, 96-103
    for water aerobics, 118-123
    for water calisthenics, 125-136
    for water exercise program, 114-117
    for water stretches, 136-143
Exercise plans. *See also* Aerobic exercise,
        program for; Muscle conditioning,
        exercise program for; Stretch exercise,
        program for; Water exercise, program
        for
    examples of, 149-157
    general guidelines for, ix-x, 6-9,
        147-148, 158 (*see also* Safety)
    and individual needs, viii-ix, 21-22
    self-motivation for, 6-7, 160-162
    starting, 6-9
Exercise risks. *See also* Medical disorders;
        Safety
    for general health, 19
    for injury, viii, 31, 38, 58, 59, 65, 94

F

Feet, exercises for, 89-90, 108-109
Fibrinogen, 14
Fingers, exercises for, 74-75, 100-101
Flexibility. *See also* Stretch exercise
    benefits of exercise for, ix, 3, 15, 17, 91,
        92, 159
    effect of aging on, 94-95
Floor surfaces in safety, 22
Forearm, exercises for, 74-75, 100-101
Frequency
    for aerobic exercise, 40, 41, 42, 112, 147
    for exercise in general, 7
    for muscle conditioning, 59, 60-61, 112,
        147
    and safety, 31
    for stretch exercise, 92, 112
    for water exercise, 112-113
Frostbite, 24

G
Gavin, James, 161
Greist, J.H., 16
Gulton, L., 16

H
Hamstrings, exercises for, 28, 83-84, 93, 103-104
Hardman, A.E., 13
Harris survey, 4
Harvard University, 6
HDL cholesterol, 13, 17
Health clubs, choosing, 22-23
Heart, 12, 13, 25. *See also* Cardiovascular disease; Circulatory system; Heart attack; Heart rate
Heart attack, 12, 13
Heart rate
  for aerobic exercise, 30, 38-40, 42, 43, 114, 158
  in warm-up/cool-down, 26, 28, 29, 114
  for weight control, 43
Heat exhaustion/stroke, 23
High blood pressure. *See* Hypertension
Humidity in safety, 23
Hyperextension, 32, 65, 95, 116
Hypertension
  and aerobics, 37, 44
  benefits of exercise for, 12, 17, 37
  and muscle conditioning, 58, 64
  and safety, 20, 21
  and stretch exercise, 93
Hyperthermia, 23
Hypothermia, 23

I
Illness. *See* Medical disorders; *specific illnesses*
Inactivity and health, 4, 14
Injury. *See also* Safety
  and the aging process, 57-58
  through exercise, viii, 31, 38, 58, 59, 65, 94
Insomnia, 16
Institute of Aerobic Research, 5
Instructors. *See* Supervision in safety
Intensity
  of aerobic exercise, 28, 38-40, 42, 43, 48, 112, 114-115, 158
  and benefits, 4-5
  and exercise safety, 30, 31, 32, 158
  and humidity, 23
  of muscle conditioning, 59, 60, 112
  and muscle soreness, 31
  of stretch exercise, 92, 112
  in warm-ups, 25-26, 27
  of water exercise, 112-113
  for weight control, 43
Irritability, 16
Isometric exercise, 58, 63-64

J
Joints. *See also* Arthritis; Musculoskeletal system
  benefits of exercise for, 14-15, 17, 37, 63
  protection for safety, 31-32, 45, 65
Journal of the American Geriatrics Society, 12

L
Leisure activity options, listed, 7
Ligaments, 14. *See also* Joints
Lungs, benefits of exercise for, 12-13

M
Medical disorders. *See also specific disorders*
  and aerobic exercise, 37, 43-44, 113
  and muscle conditioning, 58, 61-64
  and safety, 20, 21, 31
  and stretch exercise, 92-94
  and water exercise, 61, 113-114
Medication and safety, 21, 38, 93
Mental health, benefits of exercise for, 16-17, 159. *See also* Stress reduction
Metabolism, 15-16
Midsection. *See* Abdominal region, exercises for
Motivation for exercise, 6-7, 160-162
Muscle conditioning. *See also* Calisthenics
  benefits of, 57-58, 64, 65
  duration of, 59, 60, 66, 112
  exercise program for, 64-66
  exercises for abdominals in, 80-83
  exercises for arm and shoulder, 67-75
  exercises for back, 76-77
  exercises for chest, 77-79
  exercises for lower body, 83-90
  frequency for, 59, 60-61, 112, 147
  intensity of, 59, 60, 112
  with medical disorders, 61-64
  progression for, 61
  types of, 58-59
  warm-up/cool-down for, 66
Muscles. *See also* Muscle conditioning; Musculoskeletal system; Stress reduction
  benefits of exercise for, 14-15, 17, 37
  soreness of, 30-31
Musculoskeletal system. *See also* Joints; Muscle conditioning; Muscles; Stretch exercise
  effects of aging on, 14, 57-58
  general exercise benefits for, 3, 14-15, 17, 57-58, 91
  and safety, 21-22
  and specific exercise for, 37, 63, 113
Music
  for aerobic exercise, 45-46, 48, 117
  for calisthenic workouts, 65-66, 117
  and safety, 23, 117
  for self-motivation, 160

Music *(continued)*
for stretch exercise, 95
for water exercise, 117

N

National Council on Aging, 4
National Health and Nutrition
Examination Surveys, 16
Nausea, 30
Neck, exercises for, 96
Nutrition, 6, 15, 163

O

Obesity. *See* Weight control
*Older Person's Guide to Cardiovascular
Health* (American Heart Association),
37
Osteoporosis
general exercise benefits for, vii, 14
and specific exercise, 43, 61, 62, 93, 113
Overexertion, vii-viii, 30, 117. *See also*
Duration; Intensity

P

Paffenbarger, R.S., 5-6
Physical Fitness and the Older Person
(Biegel), 16
Physician, role of, 20-22, 30, 38, 64, 163
Physician and Sportsmedicine, The (Greist et
al.), 16
Pollock, M.L., 12
Pool exercise. *See* Water exercise
Posture
benefits of exercise for, 15, 17
and exercise safety, 31-32
and specific exercise, 61, 93, 116-117
Pulse rate. *See* Heart rate

Q

Quadriceps, stretch exercises for, 104, 105

R

Range of motion, defined, 91. *See also*
Flexibility
Relaxation. *See* Stress reduction
Resistance training, 59-60, 61, 62
Respiration. *See* Breathing; Circulatory
system; Lungs, benefits of exercise
for

S

Safety. *See also* Medical disorders
in aerobic exercise, 45
and exercise environment, 22-24
general guidelines for, 25-33, 158
in muscle conditioning exercise, 58, 59,
64-65
physician's role in, 20-22, 30, 38, 64,
163
shoes for, 24
stress testing for, 19-20
in stretch exercise, 91-92, 93, 94, 95
in water exercise, 23, 112, 116-117

Self-motivation for exercise, 6-7, 160-162
Senior Fitness training program (AFAA),
23
Shin, exercises for, 63, 88-89, 108-109
Shoes for safety, 24
Shortness of breath, 30
Shoulders, exercises for, 61, 67-71, 93,
97-99
Sitting down safely, 32-33
Skeletal system, benefits of exercise for,
14-15, 17, 37
Slattery, M.L., 4
Smith, E.L., 14
Sound. *See* Acoustics in safety
Standing up safely, 32
Strength. *See also* Calisthenics; Muscle
conditioning
benefits of exercise for, 3, 17, 57, 59,
159
effects of aging on, 11, 14
Stress reduction
through exercise in general, ix, 16, 17
through specific exercise, 44, 64, 94, 114
Stress testing, 19-20
Stretch exercise
benefits of, 17, 91, 93-94
duration of, 92, 94, 112
in exercise plans, 8, 148, 151-157
exercises for back and lower body,
103-109
exercises for upper body, 96-103
frequency for, 92, 112
intensity of, 92, 112
and medical disorders, 92-94
between muscle conditioning exercises,
66, 117
program for, 94-95
in warm-up/cool-down, 27, 28
warm-up for, 25-27, 28-29, 94, 95
in water, 112, 115, 117, 136-143
Stroke, 12, 13
Sunscreen, 24, 116
Supervision in safety, 23, 59
Swimming pools. *See* Water exercise

T

Temperature for exercise, 23-24, 113
Tendons, 14. *See also* Joints
Thigh, exercises for, 63, 83-84, 85-88,
104-107
Tissue plasminogen activator (TPA), 13-14
Toes, exercises for, 89-90
Topics in Geriatric Rehabilitation, 57
TPA (tissue plasminogen activator), 13-14
Triceps, exercises for, 73, 97-98
Triglycerides, 13, 17

U

University of Texas Health Science
Center, 13-14

University of Texas Lifetime Health Letter,
    41-42
University of Utah, 4
Urinary accidents, 24

V

Visibility in safety, 22
$\dot{V}O2$ capacity, 11, 12, 17, 37

W

Walking for exercise, 8, 13, 37
Warm-up/cool-down
    for aerobic exercise, 25-28, 29, 48, 114,
        116
    for muscle conditioning, 66
    for preventing muscle soreness, 31
    role of safety, 25-29
    for stretch exercise, 25-27, 28-29, 94, 95
    for water exercise, 114-115, 116
Water, drinking, 24, 116
Water exercise
    aerobics in, 43, 112-113, 114, 115, 116,
        117, 118-123
    benefits of, 43, 92, 111
    calisthenics in, 115, 117, 125-136

duration of, 112-113
in exercise plans, 8, 148, 149-157
frequency for, 112-113
intensity of, 112-113
and medical disorders, 61, 113-114
program for, 114-117
stretch exercise in, 112, 115, 117,
    136-143
temperature for, 23, 113
warm-up/cool-down for, 114-115, 116
Weight control
    through aerobic exercise, 37, 43,
        113-114
    benefits of general exercise for, vii, ix,
        3, 15-16, 17
    through muscle conditioning, 64
    through water exercise, 113-114
Weights
    beneficial use of, 60, 61, 62, 63
    harmful use of, 27, 42, 58
Wharton, M.A., 57
Wrist, exercises for, 74-75, 100-101

Y

Yoga, 91-92

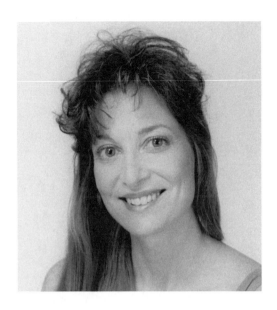

About the Author

Janie T. Clark is an exercise physiologist with an extensive background in working with mature audiences and the host of the PBS television series *The Wellness Workout*.

Janie has a master's degree in exercise physiology and wellness management from the University of Central Florida. She has served as a specialty consultant on senior fitness for the Aerobics and Fitness Association of America, helping to develop its senior fitness training program for instructors who work with older populations. She is the director of ABLE (Arthritis: Better Living through Exercise), an exercise program designed specifically for those with debilitating rheumatoid and osteoarthritis.

Janie is the author of *Seniorcise: A Simple Guide to Fitness for the Elderly and Disabled*, and *The Wellness Way*, which is the companion book for her television series. Janie is also a health and fitness instructor for Daytona Beach Community College.

Janie and her husband, Grant, live in New Smyrna Beach, Florida, along with their three cats and two dogs.